The Surgical Portfolio and Interview:

A COMPLETE GUIDE

The Surgical Portfolio and Interview:

A COMPLETE GUIDE

JOE ESLAND

BSc (Hons) MBChB (Hons) MRCSEd
Specialty Registrar in Trauma and Orthopaedic Surgery, Edinburgh Rotation
Doctoral candidate and Medical Education Fellow, University of Edinburgh

ANDREW HALL

BMedSci (Hons) MBChB MRCSEd
Specialty Registrar in Trauma and Orthopaedic Surgery, Edinburgh Rotation
Doctoral candidate and Medical Education Fellow, University of Edinburgh

Scion

© **Scion Publishing Ltd, 2021**

First published 2021

A CIP catalogue record for this book is available from the British Library.

ISBN 9781911510819

Scion Publishing Limited

The Old Hayloft, Vantage Business Park, Bloxham Road, Banbury OX16 9UX, UK

www.scionpublishing.com

Important Note from the Publisher
The information contained within this book was obtained by Scion Publishing Ltd from sources believed by us to be reliable. However, while every effort has been made to ensure its accuracy, no responsibility for loss or injury whatsoever occasioned to any person acting or refraining from action as a result of information contained herein can be accepted by the authors or publishers.

Readers are reminded that medicine is a constantly evolving science and while the authors and publishers have ensured that all dosages, applications and practices are based on current indications, there may be specific practices which differ between communities. You should always follow the guidelines laid down by the manufacturers of specific products and the relevant authorities in the country in which you are practising.

Although every effort has been made to ensure that all owners of copyright material have been acknowledged in this publication, we would be pleased to acknowledge in subsequent reprints or editions any omissions brought to our attention.

Registered names, trademarks, etc. used in this book, even when not marked as such, are not to be considered unprotected by law.

Typeset by Medlar Publishing Solutions Pvt Ltd, India

Printed in the UK

Last digit is the print number: 10 9 8 7 6 5 4 3 2 1

Contents

Preface.. ix

Acknowledgements.. xi

How to use this book..xiii

Section 1: Introduction..1

Ch 1: **A career in surgery**..3

    1.1: Direct clinical care 3

    1.2: Supporting professional activities....................................5

    1.3: Additional NHS responsibilities...5

Ch 2: **Training outline and requirements for progression**................7

    2.1: Training structure 7

    2.2: Requirements for progression 8

Section 2: The surgical portfolio.....................11

Ch 3: **Portfolio presentation and structure**.........................13

    3.1: Table of contents...14

    3.2: Structure..14

Ch 4: **Portfolio maintenance and the surgical logbook** 17

    4.1: General principles...17

    4.2: Evidence required...17

    4.3: Surgical logbook 19

Ch 5: **Creating good opportunities and maximising yield** 21

    5.1: Creating good opportunities 21

    5.2: Maximising yield...23

Ch 6: Portfolio domains 25
6.1: Using this chapter 25
6.2: Research 27
6.3: Teaching and education 30
6.4: Quality improvement and clinical audit 32
6.5: Leadership and management 35
6.6: Academic achievement and higher degrees 38
6.7: Commitment to specialty 40

Section 3: The surgical interview 43

Ch 7: General interview advice 45
7.1: Preparation 45
7.2: Interview day 46

Ch 8: Understanding the question 49
8.1: Closed questions about professional qualities 50
8.2: Open questions 50
8.3: Ethics and professionalism 51
8.4: Clinical scenarios 51
8.5: Specific knowledge 52

Ch 9: Characteristics assessed at interview – 'buzzwords' 53

Ch 10: Professional qualities 55
10.1: How to answer questions about professional qualities 55
10.2: Research 58
10.3: Teaching and education 61
10.4: Quality improvement and clinical audit 63
10.5: Leadership and management 66
10.6: Communication 69
10.7: Teamwork 72
10.8: Working under pressure 75
10.9: Probity 77
10.10: Empathy and compassion 79

Ch 11: Open questions 83
11.1: How to answer open questions 83
11.2: Why surgery? 85
11.3: Why this specialty? 87
11.4: Why this region's programme? 90
11.5: Tell me about yourself 93
11.6: What are your weaknesses? 96

Ch 12: Ethics and professionalism 99
12.1: How to answer ethics and professionalism questions 99
12.2: Common themes 101
12.3: Practice questions 109

Ch 13: Clinical scenarios 113
13.1: Purpose of this chapter 113
13.2: How to answer clinical questions 114
13.3: General surgery 117
13.4: Trauma and orthopaedic surgery 123
13.5: Vascular and cardiothoracic surgery 130
13.6: Neurosurgery 134
13.7: Plastic surgery 139
13.8: Urology 143
13.9: Ear, nose and throat surgery 146
13.10: Perioperative care 149
13.11: Advanced trauma life support (ATLS) 151
13.12: Managing a theatre list 154

Ch 14: Knowledge-based interview stations 159
14.1: Apprenticeship 159
14.1.1: Capacity 159
14.1.2: Consent 163
14.1.3: Confidentiality 169
14.1.4: Handover 171
14.1.5: Triage 173
14.1.6: Patient safety 175

14.1.7: Adverse event management... 177

14.1.8: Order of escalation... 180

14.1.9: Challenging consultations 182

14.2: Leadership 184

14.2.1: Responsibilities in the workplace...................................... 184

14.2.2: Ethical principles 185

14.3: Scholarship.. 186

14.3.1: Statistical definitions.. 186

14.3.2: Study designs... 191

14.3.3: Patient-reported outcome measures............................... 196

14.3.4: Research funding... 198

Preface

This book has been written in an attempt to prevent aspiring surgeons from unknowingly falling foul of the selection processes. This, unfortunately, is an outcome that we have observed far too often.

Every medical trainee knows that obtaining a surgical training post is competitive; however, you learn of this at a stage in your training when it is intangible. How many pre-clinical medical students can honestly say that they have started to thoughtfully curate a surgical portfolio? Yet, it is an important prerequisite to a successful application.

Section 2 of this book describes *what* you need to add to your portfolio and *how* it can be achieved. The advice is pragmatic, with particular attention given to ensuring you create opportunities that generate a proportionate return on your investment of effort and time, as well as how to gain all available credit from them. By following this guidance, the shortlisting score required to gain an interview should simply be a formality.

The surgical interview is an exam – a detail referred to many times throughout this book – but not one that you'll find a syllabus for. Unfortunately, this can lead to a preoccupation with learning the 'knowledge' for the interview, so detracting from the other important quality for performing well on the day: *your interview technique*.

Therefore, *Section 3* of this book has two purposes: first, to equip the reader – either directly or by signposting to suitable resources – with the commonly assessed interview content and, as importantly, to provide tools that you can use to improve your interview technique. We would encourage you to repeatedly utilise these tools when preparing your interview answers and practising their delivery.

If you follow the advice in this book, we are confident that you will significantly increase the likelihood of securing your desired training post. We wish you every success in that endeavour and with your future career.

Joe Esland
Andrew Hall

Acknowledgements

Joe Esland

I would like to thank my wife, Rachel, for her unwavering encouragement, support and facilitation of my time-consuming pursuits.

To my dog, Poppy, thanks for being you; your innate ability to entertain and distract has made writing this book during a pandemic an altogether more enjoyable experience.

Andrew Hall

I would like to thank those people who have been so supportive of my own surgical journey to date. Sue, my mum, is unerringly diligent and taught me that "anything is possible if you work hard enough"; Niamh is patient, encouraging, and her quiet counsel is the best support I could wish for. I'm indebted to mentors in the clinical, academic, and sporting worlds. If you think this might apply to you – it definitely does.

How to use this book

Surgery is an interesting, exciting and gratifying career, which offers a wealth of opportunities and experiences that are unique to the profession. It is founded upon a deep understanding of anatomy and pathology – with which you'll be familiar – but, in the acquisition of surgical competencies, doctors must develop a new set of knowledge and skills that are distinct from their prior medical training. **You therefore have to work very hard to obtain the rewards that the career offers.**

Portfolio

Modern methods of candidate selection are seemingly predicated on this point. Simply put, you must show, throughout all stages of your medical training, that you have an outstanding work ethic and achieve highly. If you fail in this endeavour, you will not be selected for interview. This invariably leads to disappointment, years out to bolster your CV and perhaps a change in career.

In *Section 2* of this book we will explain how, by **thoughtfully** selecting opportunities and diligently **ensuring you gain all available credit** from them, you can meet this essential standard. The common pitfalls and mistakes made by candidates will also be described, to help avoid poor output from low quality activities. By following these simple instructions, and so curating a robust academic portfolio, you will put yourself ahead and make shortlisting for interview a formality.

Interview

The surgical 'interview' is not an interview at all; it is an exam. Unfortunately, this is not well appreciated, and we have seen many outstanding junior colleagues perform poorly at interview due to this oversight. Your interview score will be related to your ability to answer in a structured manner, mention the 'buzzwords' and have good foundational knowledge; helpfully, the questions are relatively predictable.

A significant part of this book is therefore dedicated to preparing you for the interview, covering the most commonly questioned themes, and providing structured methods for answering comprehensively. If you learn the content of this book, prepare your answers as described and practise their delivery using the structures provided, you can excel and score highly.

We have provided you with a number of acronyms, for example ROSES and OPALS, that can be used to help you prepare your answers. These are presented consistently throughout the book and you can find them all in full on the inside front cover where they can easily be referred to while practising interview answers.

Use this book as an instruction manual

It is our hope that you use this book as an instruction manual and it is therefore written as such, with strong recommendations made throughout. Of course, that is not to say that the instructions provided herein are the only way of scoring well; they are simply a reliable means of doing so.

If you follow our advice, we are confident that you will significantly increase the likelihood of securing your desired training post.

Section 1:

1

Introduction

Ch 1: A career in surgery 3

    1.1: Direct clinical care 3

    1.2: Supporting professional activities 5

    1.3: Additional NHS responsibilities 5

Ch 2: Training outline and requirements for progression 7

    2.1: Training structure 7

    2.2: Requirements for progression 8

CHAPTER 1:

A career in surgery

The requirements of a surgical Consultant are broad, encompassing not just clinical capabilities, but also a vast breadth of **non-clinical requirements and optional opportunities**. We include this section to describe these requirements – as set out by Consultants' contracts and medical governing bodies – to illustrate why you, as an applicant, are required to demonstrate many of the characteristics laid out in this book. It is hoped that by understanding this from the outset it will enable the reader to write more meaningful answers, based on a better appreciation of their future role.

1.1: Direct clinical care

This is the most obvious requirement of a Consultant and is based on the syllabuses published by the Intercollegiate Surgical Curriculum Programme (ISCP; www.iscp.ac.uk/curriculum/surgical/surgical_syllabus_list.aspx), which sets out the clinical knowledge and skills required to complete the training programme (CCT – Certificate of Completion of Training).

Many of the characteristics necessary to provide excellent clinical care are needed at all levels of training, although the requirement for competence in leadership and management increases with time. **These clinical requirements are set out plainly in *Good Medical Practice*** published by the General Medical Council (GMC, 2013) and can be summarised as follows:

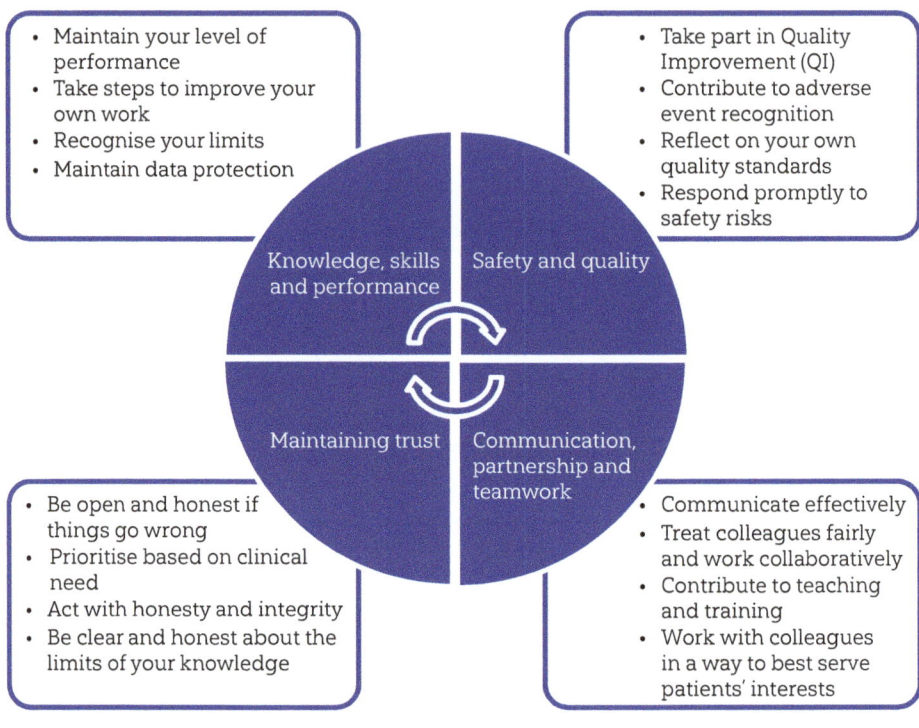

- Maintain your level of performance
- Take steps to improve your own work
- Recognise your limits
- Maintain data protection

- Take part in Quality Improvement (QI)
- Contribute to adverse event recognition
- Reflect on your own quality standards
- Respond promptly to safety risks

Knowledge, skills and performance

Safety and quality

Maintaining trust

Communication, partnership and teamwork

- Be open and honest if things go wrong
- Prioritise based on clinical need
- Act with honesty and integrity
- Be clear and honest about the limits of your knowledge

- Communicate effectively
- Treat colleagues fairly and work collaboratively
- Contribute to teaching and training
- Work with colleagues in a way to best serve patients' interests

With this in mind, remember that interviewers are **not** solely looking at a candidate's potential to fulfil the technical requirements of the training programme. Although this is clearly an important factor, **excellent surgeons are also outstanding in the many other areas of clinical practice.**

Resource: Non-technical skills for surgeons (NOTSS)

NOTSS describes the main non-technical skills observed in theatre that contribute to good surgical practice. It describes four domains:
- situational awareness
- decision-making
- communication and teamwork
- leadership.

More can be found here: www.rcsed.ac.uk/media/415471/notss-handbook-2012.pdf

---

1.2: Supporting professional activities

These are set out in the job plan of a Consultant, with commonly included commitments stated in the table below. Broadly, these activities have the intention of **improving the quality and safety of patient care**.

Additional supporting activities of a Consultant	
Medical education	Research
Training	Management
Formal teaching	Appraisal
Quality improvement	Job planning
Clinical audit	Clinical governance

Many Consultants will take on **substantive roles** within the above areas, for which they are directly responsible, and are given time within their job plans to allow them to fulfil the requirements of the post. This emphasises the importance of the prospective trainee's need to demonstrate aptitude in areas such as education, training, quality improvement and research.

1.3: Additional NHS responsibilities

Some Consultants will take on additional **managerial** positions, although this is not an absolute requirement; however, with the current trend in healthcare management leaning towards greater involvement of clinicians in decision-making, it seems reasonable to suggest that these roles will increase in number and importance.

Current examples include Clinical Director, Training Programme Director, Clinical Audit Lead, and Undergraduate or Postgraduate Dean.

Application and interview scoring now typically awards the equivalent number of points for leadership / management achievements as for research / audit / teaching. **It is important that this area of professional development is not overlooked.**

Reference

General Medical Council (2013) *Good Medical Practice*. Available at: https://www.gmc-uk.org/ethical-guidance/ethical-guidance-for-doctors/good-medical-practice

Introduction

CHAPTER 2:

Training outline and requirements for progression

An appreciation of the training structure and the annual requirements for progression demonstrates commitment to surgical training.

2.1: Training structure

Surgical training takes between seven and eight years. Most programmes are 'uncoupled', meaning that there are two selection processes over this time; first, for entry into Core Training (CT1–2) and, secondly, into Specialty Training (ST3–8). Broadly then, there are two routes for entry into a surgical training programme:

1. Entry into ST1 'run-through' training after the successful completion of FY2
2. Entry into ST3 training after the completion of CT2

The current exceptions to this are described in the table below.

Specialties which do not follow the 'uncoupled' structure	
Specialty	Training structure
Neurosurgery	All of these programmes are either (i) 'run-through' from ST1–8, without an application at ST3 or (ii) 'uncoupled', but have specialty-specific requirements for entry into ST3
Oral and maxillofacial	
Cardiothoracics	
Orthopaedics (in Scotland only)	'Run-through' from ST1–8

Resource: Joint Committee on Surgical Training (JCST): *Intercollegiate Surgical Curriculum Programme* (ISCP; www.iscp.ac.uk)

It is important to note that this training structure is changing from August 2021. Broadly, however, the selection points for entry into training are similar.

This has been driven by a change in the surgical curriculum and methods of assessment.

Full details on this, including the new specialty-specific curricula, training pathways and training duration, can be found here: www.iscp.ac.uk/iscp/curriculum-2021

Please note: the requirements for progression, described in *Section 2.2* (below), are therefore also likely to change.

2.2: Requirements for progression

Annually, surgical trainees are required to attend a meeting to confirm that they are making progress at the expected rate – this is termed the **Annual Review of Competence Progression** (ARCP). All of your achievements are evidenced using two resources, which are maintained and updated regularly:
- The ISCP Portfolio (www.ISCP.ac.uk)
- The surgical eLogbook (www.eLogbook.org)

2.2.1: ISCP portfolio

The portfolio is a record of your achievements throughout the year and, importantly, is also where all of your work-based assessments are recorded. Many of the requirements are familiar and include:
- procedure-based assessments (PBAs), clinical evaluation exercises (CEX), direct observation of procedural skills (DOPS), case-based discussions (CBD), multi-source feedback (MSF) and others; **there is a minimum number of these which must be completed each year**
- passing mandatory examinations
- audit and QI
- research and other publications (e.g. book chapters)
- attendance at conferences and courses
- awards and prizes
- teaching sessions
- positions of responsibility
- reflective practice.

2.2.2: Surgical eLogbook

See *Section 4.3* for detailed information on maintaining your surgical logbook. This is a real-time record of your operative experience and includes every procedure that you have been involved in, whether as primary surgeon, assistant or observer. **It can be started as a medical student**; however, only procedures from ST3 onwards count towards your final 'numbers'. You must meet the minimum number of operations annually and over the training programme as a whole.

> ### Exams: Member of the Royal College of Surgeons (MRCS)
>
> The MRCS examination contains two parts: Part A is a written component and Part B is a clinical exam. **Both Part A and Part B must be completed before the end of CT2/ST2 to allow progression into ST3.** You can sit the exam at any point after medical school.

Section 2:

2

The surgical portfolio

Ch 3: Portfolio presentation and structure 13

    3.1: Table of contents 14

    3.2: Structure 14

Ch 4: Portfolio maintenance and the surgical logbook 17

    4.1: General principles 17

    4.2: Evidence required 17

    4.3: Surgical logbook 19

Ch 5: Creating good opportunities and maximising yield 21

    5.1: Creating good opportunities 21

    5.2: Maximising yield 23

Ch 6: Portfolio domains 25

    6.1: Using this chapter 25

    6.2: Research 27

    6.3: Teaching and education 30

    6.4: Quality improvement and clinical audit 32

    6.5: Leadership and management 35

    6.6: Academic achievement and higher degrees 38

    6.7: Commitment to specialty 40

CHAPTER 3:

Portfolio presentation and structure

In these next few pages we refer to the **physical, hard copy** of your portfolio that you are asked to produce at interview. The contents of this chapter may therefore seem obvious; however, portfolios are not often well presented and are **typically awarded points** towards your overall application score. A well-presented portfolio is therefore worth the effort! There is no gold standard but the table below describes some recommendations.

Feature	Recommendations
Folder	• An A4 ring binder in a neutral colour • Consider personalising it with your name on the cover
Pages	• All single-sided, where possible • Every page contained within an individual, good quality plastic cover • Consider marking / highlighting pertinent information on a page. For example, if you've presented your work at a conference, and you include the acceptance email, highlight the text within the email that confirms the meeting name, date, their acceptance and the type of presentation (e.g. poster or podium)
Indexing	• Mark the top right-hand corner of each page with a page number – you can buy these as stickers, which you then apply • Keep the pages in order
Sections	• Use different coloured section dividers to keep all relevant material together • Ensure that section dividers are labelled legibly and clearly

3.1: Table of contents

Write a table of contents and keep this at the front of your portfolio. Within each section, put your most impressive achievements first (and thus the ones that will score you most marks). Put the remainder in order of importance. As an example:

Clinical Audit and Quality Improvement	
Aug 2016	*Improving Compliance with National Guidance in the Management of Neck of Femur Fractures* Presented at the national Hip Fracture Symposium – 1st Prize
Apr 2018	*Peer-Assisted Learning for Foundation Doctors in a Major Trauma Centre* Presented at the regional Quality Improvement meeting
Nov 2014	*An Audit of Neuro-observations Following Head Injury* Presented at the Emergency Department Grand Round

3.2: Structure

There is no single best way to structure your portfolio: a logical, easy-to-follow layout is all that is necessary, although there are some broadly accepted standards. Below, we provide a recommended structure.

1. Table of contents
2. Curriculum vitae (x3)
3. Qualifications
   - This should include your GMC registration, your medical degree and any other higher qualifications
4. Academic achievement and prizes
5. Courses
6. Research
7. Quality improvement and clinical audit
8. Teaching and training
9. Leadership and management

10. Conferences
11. Surgical logbook
12. Surgical experience
    • This should include postgraduate 'taster weeks', undergraduate surgical experience and any other surgical exposure
13. Professional memberships
14. Reflective practice

Note, this is a generic layout; however, some interviews will require you to format your portfolio in a specified format. Ensure you follow the instructions strictly.

CHAPTER 4:

Portfolio maintenance and the surgical logbook

As a surgical trainee, your portfolio is prospectively maintained throughout the year, and the evidence you must record is orders of magnitude more extensive than at any prior stage of training. It is therefore very reasonable for interviewers to expect that applicants have also maintained their portfolio to a high standard.

4.1: General principles

- **Prospectively** maintain your portfolio from the earliest possible time at medical school – you will never regret having 'too much' evidence in your portfolio.
  - If you forget to evidence something, retrospectively contact your supervisor.
- For each project you complete, you should **ask your supervisor for a letter**:
  - describing the project and its importance
  - stating your personal contribution to its success.
- Keep all evidence as a **physical** copy, where possible, as most interviews will require you to submit a 'hard copy' of your portfolio.
  - All paperwork should be **single-sided**, if possible.

4.2: Evidence required

In addition to a letter (described above) the other evidence required is as follows:

Activity	Evidence
Academic performance	• Academic transcript • Degree certificates
GMC registration	• Your original GMC certificate
Prizes and scholarships	• A letter / email from the awarding body
Publications	• A copy of the manuscript • A letter / email from the journal confirming acceptance • PubMed ID (PMID)
Presentations	• A printed copy of the presentation, 4–6 slides per page • A letter / email from the meeting confirming acceptance and if a podium or poster presentation
Courses	• A certificate of completion
Conferences	• A certificate of attendance
Audit and QI	• A copy of the manuscript • A printed copy of the **initial** presentation, 4–6 slides per page • A printed copy of the **second cycle** presentation, 4–6 slides per page • A letter confirming where it was presented
SSCs	• A letter from the administrative team at your medical school, confirming completion of the SSC
Taster weeks	• A letter from the supervising Consultant
Reflective practice	• Short reflective essays
Professional memberships	• Confirmation email of membership • Your membership number
Miscellaneous	• A letter from your supervisor

4.3: Surgical logbook

In the UK, your surgical logbook should be maintained using www.elogbook.org.

This is the gold standard and is recommended by many of the specialty colleges, including orthopaedics, neurosurgery, urology, ENT and plastics.

For each case, you should input the following data:
- Patient ID
- Patient age
- NCEPOD grade: elective, scheduled, urgent or emergency (see *Section 14.1.5*, Triage)
- ASA grade
- Responsible Consultant
- Supervision level: observed, supervised-trainer scrubbed (STS), supervised-trainer unscrubbed (STU) or performed
- Operation name
- Hospital
- Any specific notes about the case

CHAPTER 5:

Creating good opportunities and maximising yield

In this chapter, we will explain the principles of:
- how to create excellent opportunities
- how to maximise the points you accrue from each opportunity.

An understanding of these principles will help to avoid the many pitfalls that students and junior doctors often fall into when undertaking these activities; most commonly, spending too much time on a pursuit that never had a realistic prospect of offering a return.

Simply put, it is better to undertake a single project that fulfils the criteria set out below, rather than undertake multiple poor quality, low yield projects.

5.1: Creating good opportunities

We use the term 'opportunity' to describe any pursuit that will score marks in the surgical application and interview.

1. **You created and designed it**

   Although it might seem unrealistic at first, creating and designing opportunities is perfectly achievable, irrespective of your stage of training. In areas such as teaching, education, audit, quality improvement, leadership and management, you need little experience to create and design a project.

   The most common apprehension candidates express is the lack of a 'novel' idea; however, this is not what is required. Instead, **look for things that are already successful and try to improve them**.

2. Pertinent to the specialty

Whilst this is not an absolute requirement, it is always preferable to undertake opportunities in the future specialty that you plan to apply for. It will get your face known locally and this then tends to help create further opportunities down the line. Furthermore, it will improve your understanding and insight into the specialty, giving you valuable content that you can discuss at interview.

3. A regular commitment for >3–6 months

In general, opportunities you undertake should require a regular commitment for a minimum of 3–6 months. This is especially important for leadership and management roles, where the time commitment will specifically score you marks.

4. Time commitment is proportional to its value

It is essential that you feel the time commitment required to complete a project is proportional to the value it adds to your CV. For example, you might spend many hours on a novel research project with the expectation of a first-author paper in a peer-reviewed journal; however, the same time commitment spent on an audit which is then presented at the local departmental meeting would represent a poor opportunity.

The caveat to this statement is that, if you've not much else going on, it is still preferable to undertake a project that offers a poor return on your time, rather than doing nothing at all.

5. Clear outcomes and targets

There should be an expectation that all work is presented or published. Therefore, from the outset there should be clear, explicit expectations for the work; in particular, the level of meeting or journal that you are aiming for. Furthermore, understanding this from the beginning will help avoid disappointment due to a mismatch between your expectations and those of your collaborators.

6. Provides scope to meet multiple assessment criteria

By following the above criteria, it is possible to score well within many separate domains by undertaking a single project. In particular, points in 'leadership' and 'commitment to specialty' can be easily met through most opportunities.

5.2: Maximising yield

To ensure that you maximise the points you accrue from every opportunity, you should try to meet the criteria below.

1. **Completed**

   You should not start a project if you cannot realistically complete it within the time frame you have available; you do not score marks for incomplete work and, worse, it is an unfavourable trait to present at interview.

   This is one of the most common mistakes made by applicants.

2. **Presented**

   Ensure that all work you undertake is presented, in some form, at a meeting or conference. There is a wealth of meetings at all levels – whether departmental, regional or national – and you should have an expectation that your work is presented somewhere.

   Furthermore, presenting at meetings is a good way to network and is an opportunity to gain academic prizes.

3. **Recognised**

   Ensure that you have your contribution formally recognised, ideally in a letter, by the most senior person that was involved. Practically, this would usually mean that you draft a letter outlining your contribution and send it to the supervisor, so that they can then amend it and return it to you. Keep all of these letters in your professional portfolio; **they will all be required as evidence of your achievements during interview.**

4. **Formal feedback**

   You should aim to appraise your performance regularly, particularly in teaching and leadership. There are freely accessible, validated appraisal tools that you can hand out to gain feedback. Collate the data and file this in your portfolio, as it is a favourable trait of an applicant and will be useful to talk about at interview.

5. **Reflected upon**

   Following the completion of all substantial projects, try to complete a reflective piece of work. This may score you marks in your application but, importantly, it provides insightful experiences that you can discuss at interview.

CHAPTER 6:

Portfolio domains

6.1: Using this chapter

The sections within this chapter address the domains that are assessed in the surgical portfolio and are therefore **responsible for your shortlisting score**. These domains are:

- Research (*Section 6.2*)
- Teaching and education (*Section 6.3*)
- Quality improvement and clinical audit (*Section 6.4*)
- Leadership and management (*Section 6.5*)
- Academic achievements and higher degrees (*Section 6.6*)
- Commitment to specialty (*Section 6.7*).

The intention of this chapter is to demonstrate how you can achieve maximum marks in each domain, as well as to illustrate how you can use these achievements to perform well at interview.

Each section is written following the same structured format and, over the next few pages, the pedagogical features utilised are described.

Golden rules

Every page begins by describing the 'golden rules' that should be adhered to when undertaking an opportunity within that domain. These have been collated by assessing the scoring systems for various surgical applications (such as core surgical training and specialty run-through programmes) to identify the common themes. By fulfilling these criteria, you will maximise the points you accrue for every opportunity that you complete.

6.1.1: Skills demonstrated

The transferable skills – usually referred to as 'buzzwords' – that are developed by undertaking an opportunity are shown in the three groups in the table below. These are included to help you understand the characteristics that you'll be demonstrating when you later describe these achievements, often in 'white space' questions (on an application form) or at interview.

Skills can be divided into three groups:

Apprenticeship ❯	Leadership ❯❯	Scholarship ❯❯❯
Relating to your clinical duties	Relating to your leadership and management abilities	Relating to your academic performance, in research, quality improvement and clinical audit

6.1.2: Relevance to surgical training

The purpose of completing opportunities in the portfolio domains is to develop transferable skills that will help you excel as a surgical trainee. That relationship is described in this chapter, with the hope that it will give you better insight and subsequently allow you to write more meaningful interview answers.

6.1.3: Getting started

In this chapter, some of the most common activities that often result in good opportunities being created are described. They are subdivided into 'undergraduate' and 'postgraduate', although there is of course some overlap between them.

6.1.4: Example opportunities

The common opportunities that will score you points in your surgical portfolio are described in the table below. They are categorised into good, better and best, with the latter scoring the highest number of marks.

Good ★★★	Better ★★★★	Best ★★★★★
Published in a non-peer-reviewed journal	A publication in a peer-reviewed journal, but not first-author	First-author publication in a peer-reviewed journal of original work
1st-class BMedSci	A 2.1-class intercalated BSc or MPhil	A PhD, MD or 1st-class intercalated BSc
Research presented at local meeting	A poster presentation at a national/international meeting	An oral presentation at a national/international meeting

6.1.5: Maximising yield

Maximising 'yield' relates to how you score the maximum number of marks for every opportunity you complete. The broad principles of how that is accomplished are described in *Section 5.2*.

Those principles are applied here to give you concrete examples of what you should be aiming to achieve.

> **Common pitfalls**
>
> There are many common mistakes within each domain that students and junior doctors frequently make, often leading to poor scoring despite a heavy time commitment. This is largely due to inexperience and they are therefore highlighted in this box.

6.1.6: Resources

Some useful resources will be included here.

6.2: Research

> **Golden rules**
>
> An **original** piece of research that can be **completed within the time frame** available to you. The work must have **clear scope for presentation or publication**, and you must ensure that your position in the **authorship is well defined** from the outset.

6.2.1: Skills demonstrated

Apprenticeship ❯	Leadership ❯❯	Scholarship ❯❯❯
Detail-oriented	Committed	Conscientious
Inquisitive	Communicative	Critical thinking
Organised		Disciplined
		Self-directed

6.2.2: Relevance to surgical training

Gaining competence in performing and appraising research is **essential for professional development** and the advancement of surgical practice: it is a core tenet of a surgeon's **commitment to lifelong learning**. Surgical registrars are **required to publish** research to complete their training.

6.2.3: Getting started

Undergraduate
- Look to undertake a 'student selected component' (SSC) in surgery, as this will often involve undertaking a piece of research.
- Email your local Surgical Society to ask if they've any available research projects or contacts.
- Speak with your Registrar whilst on placement – they invariably need another pair of hands!
- Consider an intercalated BSc (in surgery).

Postgraduate
- Contact the research-active Consultants and Registrars within the specialty that you're interested in.
- Look for opportunities to get involved in national collaborative research projects, which often require a local lead to collect data.
- Attend Journal Club and consider going on courses / conferences to improve your abilities.
- Consider an MD or PhD.

6.2.4: Example opportunities

Good ★★★	Better ★★★★	Best ★★★★★
Published in a non-peer-reviewed journal	A publication in a peer-reviewed journal, but not first-author	First-author publication in a peer-reviewed journal of original work
1st-class BMedSci	A 2.1-class intercalated BSc or MPhil	A PhD, MD or 1st-class intercalated BSc
Research presented at local meeting	A poster presentation at a national / international meeting	An oral presentation at a national / international meeting

6.2.5: Maximising yield

- Ensure that you are working with a team that have a **proven track record** in publishing research – look them up on a research database to see how frequently they're publishing and the journals they're commonly published in.
- Assist with **data collection and analysis**. Familiarise yourself with the commonly used statistical software, such as SPSS and Prism.
- **Identify early** the meetings / conferences that you could present your work at and ensure that **your timeline works towards these dates**.
- **Look to see if different aspects of the research can be presented at different meetings / conferences.** For example, you may wish to present some of the data at a few student conferences or local meetings, and the 'finished' work at a large specialty conference.
- Aim to present your work at an **international** conference (N.B. this doesn't necessarily mean that the conference is overseas, just that the delegates are from an international audience).
- Ensure that the journal you're publishing in has a **PubMed ID (PMID)** – these publications score higher marks in the application.

Common pitfalls

- **Not saying 'no'** to projects – if it doesn't offer a good return on the time investment, don't do it!
- Not understanding your place in the authorship order
- Failing to plan where you will present your work ahead of time – it is not uncommon for people to have spent an enormous amount of time on a research project, **but it wasn't presented / published *prior* to applications**
- Taking on **too many** projects and not completing / presenting / publishing them

The surgical portfolio

6.2.6: Resources

1. Biomedical Vacation Scholarships (https://wellcome.ac.uk/funding/schemes/biomedical-vacation-scholarships)
2. e-Learning for Healthcare – research modules (www.e-lfh.org.uk/programmes/research-audit-and-quality-improvement/)
3. National Trainee Research Collaboratives (www.asit.org/resources/national-trainee-research-collaboratives/trainee-research-collaboratives/res1137)

6.3: Teaching and education

> **Golden rules**
>
> The most essential requirement is an **ongoing commitment** to teaching and to ensure that it is **formally recognised**. To maximise scoring, **involvement in curriculum design and delivery** is key.

6.3.1: Skills demonstrated

Apprenticeship >	Leadership >>	Scholarship >>>
Communicative	Conscientious	Determined
Productive	Innovative	Motivated
	Organised	Organised
	Self-directed	

6.3.2: Relevance to surgical training

Surgical trainees are central to the ongoing training of juniors and often deliver formal departmental teaching for FY doctors. It is important to develop these skills to ensure that you're a competent trainer in both the academic and clinical settings.

6.3.3: Getting started

Undergraduate
- Contact your student Surgical Society to look for peer-assisted learning opportunities.
- Contact your medical school faculty to express an interest in peer-assisted learning.

- Set up a student specialist-interest group.
- Look for community outreach projects.

Postgraduate
- Engage in regular clinical teaching for undergraduates.
- Contact the departmental clinical lead who is responsible for undergraduate and/or FY teaching.
- Look for substantive education posts within the local medical school.
- Consider a postgraduate certificate in medical education (PGCME).

6.3.4: Example opportunities

Good ★★★	Better ★★★★	Best ★★★★★
Frequent, informal surgical teaching to juniors and peers	Office holder in a surgical society	Organising and delivering a student course or conference
Undergraduate bedside teaching	Teaching / facilitating on a course	Higher education qualification
	Regular teaching with formal feedback, collected over time	Substantive university post in education and training

6.3.5: Maximising yield

- If you have colleagues in other institutions, liaise with them to try to **implement your programme there, too**; this then makes your programme national, which increases scoring.
- **Apply for funding**, which could be used to fund local speakers or pay for workshop materials. Many places will have a small pot of money put aside for educational purposes. A good place to start is your Student Union, medical school or medical industry.
- Approach your institution to gain **formal recognition** (in the form of a headed letter) of your contribution to education and training.
- Gain **regular formal feedback** (quantitative and qualitative) before and after your teaching – there are many validated questionnaires that are freely available for this purpose. Ensure you write a reflective entry in your portfolio about how you've used this feedback for self-improvement.

The surgical portfolio

- **Present the details of your teaching / education programme** at a meeting, such as the Association for the Study of Medical Education (ASME) or Developing Excellence in Medical Education Conference (DEMEC).
- **Broaden the audience** by involving diverse groups, such as students from a local medical school or different year groups.
- Attend an **educational conference** (e.g. ASME Annual General Meeting or DEMEC).

> **Common pitfalls**
>
> - A high number of hours of **unevidenced** local teaching
> - Failure to gain formal **feedback**
> - Focusing on a single teaching modality only

6.3.6: Resources

1. Association of Surgeons in Training (ASiT)
2. eLearning for Healthcare (e-LfH) – Educator hub
3. Junior Association for the Study of Medical Education (JASME)
4. Local 'Clinical Educator' programmes

6.4: Quality improvement and clinical audit

> **Golden rules**
>
> An original piece of work that is undertaken using the **correct methodologies**. It is *essential* that it is **'closed loop'**; this means that the changes to practice that you recommend are **implemented**, and their **impact is assessed** in a second cycle. **Present the work** formally at a meeting or conference.

6.4.1: Skills demonstrated

Apprenticeship >	Leadership >>	Scholarship >>>
Professional	Committed	Analytical
Reflective	Detail oriented	High standards
Self-improving	Innovative	Motivated
	Inquisitive	

6.4.2: Quality improvement vs. clinical audit

Quality improvement (QI) describes a set of techniques that can be used to improve healthcare quality through systematic assessment and intervention. There are six 'dimensions' of quality that can be improved:

- *Safe:* avoiding harm to patients (*no needless deaths*)
- *Effective:* evidence-based care delivering benefit (*no needless pain or suffering*)
- *Person-centred:* builds service around patient (*no helplessness in those served or serving*)
- *Timely:* care delivered without harmful delay (*no unwanted waiting*)
- *Efficient:* cost-effective and without avoidable waste (*no waste*)
- *Equitable:* care that is fair to all patients and service users (*no-one left out*)

Clinical audit is simply a subtype of QI, where there is a **specific, exacting, measurable** *clinical* **'standard'**, and you look to see if the clinical standard is being met. For example, 'all patients have an MRSA swab taken within 24 hours of admission' or 'all patients with a head injury receive hourly neuro-observations'.

QI projects tend to be patient-centred and have a broad scope, without a specific, exacting clinical standard. Examples might include, 'improving patient experience in the vascular outpatient department' or 'improving the effectiveness of Hospital at Night (HAN) handover'.

6.4.3: Relevance to surgical training

QI is a vital aspect of all modern healthcare systems and is pervasive throughout every specialty. Due to increasing resource and population pressures, **the healthcare service now faces delivering safe, effective care within an increasingly challenging context**. We are well placed as clinicians to assist with this effort and, therefore, there is a **requirement** that all surgical trainees perform at least one QI project / clinical audit per year.

6.4.4: Getting started

Undergraduate

- Look to undertake an SSC that involves performing a QI project – these are becoming increasingly common in the undergraduate curriculum.
- Speak to FYs and SpRs whilst on placement; they are regularly undertaking QI projects and are often grateful for the help.

The surgical portfolio

Postgraduate

- Whilst working as an FY, **look for areas of practice that could be better within your unit**. FYs are very well placed to notice these issues, particularly on the wards. Take your ideas to the SpR or Consultant.
- Most units have a Consultant who is the departmental lead for QI; contact them and ask if you can help with any of the ongoing projects.
- Complete **eLearning** on QI and clinical audit.
- Attend a QI course or conference.

6.4.5: Example opportunities

Good ★★★	Better ★★★★	Best ★★★★★
Demonstrated knowledge of QI principles	Attended a QI course	Completed a QI fellowship, or similar
Participated in a local improvement group	Participated in a regional / national improvement group	Publication or presentation of your work
Involvement in a closed loop audit or QI project	Led a local closed loop audit or QI project	Led a regional / national closed loop audit or QI project

6.4.6: Maximising yield

- Seek QI projects and clinical audits that are:
  - **focused** (address one specific issue)
  - **useful** (are likely to change practice)
  - **deliverable** (at least one full cycle) in a short period of time.
- Look for topics in which there is **departmental interest**, as such projects are more likely to have 'buy-in' from the Consultants and management. This might mean that your recommendations for change are more readily adopted.
- Aim to **present your work** at regional or national meetings. As QI is a hot topic in medicine currently, there are plenty of well-attended meetings available, often with prizes available.

Common pitfalls

- Pursuing projects **without a predetermined goal** or purpose
- 'Picking up' low quality work that has been left uncompleted by another (N.B. conversely, high quality projects requiring completing may represent 'low hanging fruit')
- **Failing to use correct methodology** to complete your projects
- **Failing to complete a second cycle** to 'close the loop'; projects that are not closed loop do not score in the application

6.4.7: Resources

1. Agency for Healthcare Research and Quality (www.ahrq.gov)
2. Clinical Audit Support Centre (www.clinicalauditsupport.com)
3. Healthcare Quality Improvement Partnership (HQIP; www.hqip.org.uk/resource/elearning-area/#.YAQolVP7SqA)

6.5: Leadership and management

Golden rules

Leadership and management are related, but fundamentally different, entities; ensure you understand the difference and create opportunities to develop **in both**.

Leadership and management are core values and behaviours that all clinicians should develop throughout their training. Competence in these areas is assessed throughout surgical careers and *there is a trend towards developing all doctors as clinical leaders*. This is reflected in the increasing emphasis placed on its assessment.

Michael West (King's Fund) provides the following descriptions:
- Leadership: "Creates direction, alignment and commitment"
- Management: "Supporting, resourcing and facilitating day to day work".

6.5.1: Skills demonstrated

Leader		
Apprenticeship ❯	**Leadership** ❯❯	**Scholarship** ❯❯❯
Enthusiastic	Communicative	Motivated
Resilient	Negotiating	Driven to improve
Adaptable		

Manager		
Apprenticeship ❯	**Leadership** ❯❯	**Scholarship** ❯❯❯
Empathy	Communication	Attention to detail
Prioritisation	Team player	

6.5.2: Relevance to surgical training

Effective leadership and management skills are not confined to those with aspirations to take senior management roles. All clinicians operate within systems / organisations and these values are important in order to provide effective and cohesive services. Surgeons will find themselves calling upon these skills on a daily basis: as members of ward or shift teams; when providing an on-call service; on surgical firms; in outpatient or procedural clinics, and in operating theatres.

6.5.3: Getting started

Undergraduate
- Apply for local leadership roles; these are often plentiful at university and are an excellent stepping stone to more prestigious appointments.
- Apply for **membership of the Faculty of Medical Leadership and Management (FMLM)**.
- Look for roles involved with **organisation of a medical / surgical event** (e.g. a course or conference), as these will allow you to begin developing skills in management.

Postgraduate

- Look for regional / national roles in leadership. There are many varied roles that involve the representation of junior doctors on committees and societies.
- Attend **specialty conferences and courses** in leadership and management.

6.5.4: Example opportunities

Good ★★★	Better ★★★★	Best ★★★★★
Working in a multiprofessional team	Organisation of local clinical activities (e.g. educational programme, multidisciplinary team (MDT) meetings, conferences)	Leadership and management course attendance
Supervision of junior staff in audit, QI and research	Membership of the FMLM	Fellowship of the FMLM
Leadership or management role in a local / undergraduate society	Leadership or management role in a regional / postgraduate organisation	Leadership or management role in a national organisation

6.5.5: Maximising yield

- Yield in leadership and management tends to come from **your experiences whilst in post**. It is therefore essential that you maintain a portfolio of your experiences, putting particular focus on times you've dealt with complexity, interpersonal challenges within the team and managing austere environments. These provide excellent topics for discussion in interviews.
- Ensure that the committee / society provide you with **a letter confirming your post, the responsibilities thereof** and **your personal contribution**.

The surgical portfolio

Common pitfalls

- Thinking you're only able to demonstrate capabilities in leadership and management by securing a 'top' position; you can demonstrate these skills at any level of training
- Failing to understand the difference between leadership and management
- Not appreciating the need to demonstrate progression throughout your roles
- Failure to demonstrate effective leadership and management in a *collaborative* context.

6.5.6: Resources

1. FMLM: *Leadership and Management Standards for Medical Professionals*. www.fmlm. ac.uk/standards
2. GMC: *Leadership and Management for All Doctors*. www.gmc-uk.org/ethical-guidance/ ethical-guidance-for-doctors/leadership-and-management-for-all-doctors
3. NHS Healthcare Leadership Model. www.leadershipacademy.nhs.uk/resources/ healthcare-leadership-model/

6.6: Academic achievement and higher degrees

Golden rules

Recognise that demonstrating academic excellence throughout the medical degree, as well as having your scholarship recognised through **awards conferred outside the medical school**, is highly beneficial to your future career.

6.6.1: Skills demonstrated

Apprenticeship >	Leadership >>	Scholarship >>>
High standards	Conscientious	Self-directed
Intelligence	Planning	Disciplined

6.6.2: Relevance to surgical training

An ongoing commitment to high attainment is essential to ensure surgical trainees progress towards clinical excellence. Trainees manage high-stake clinical scenarios on a regular basis and their decisions must be grounded upon solid foundational understanding and knowledge.

6.6.3: Getting started

Undergraduate
- Ensure you are well prepared for each examination, aiming for **merits and distinctions**.
- **Understand how your decile is calculated** and aim to **graduate with honours**.
- Identify bursaries or scholarships available to you early: there are many available throughout your training, **especially during your intercalated BSc, your elective or if you're attending a conference abroad.**
- Keep your eye out for **prizes available to undergraduates**, especially from the surgical colleges. These are often in the form of written essays or podium presentations.
- Consider an intercalated BSc and aim to achieve a **first-class honours**.

Postgraduate
- Identify prizes available through the surgical colleges and apply for these.
- Attend **specialty conferences** – there are often many prizes available.
- Consider an **Academic Foundation Programme**. Although it doesn't gain more marks alone, it may offer better opportunities that will improve your portfolio.
- Consider taking time out to undertake an MSc, MD or PhD.

6.6.4: Example opportunities

Good ★★★	Better ★★★★	Best ★★★★★
Gaining a scholarship or bursary	Graduating with Honours	National prize in surgery
Single merit, distinction or local prize	Multiple merits, distinctions or local prizes	Higher education qualification
An intercalated BMedSci	MSc or 2.1 in an (intercalated) BSc	First-class BSc, MD or PhD

6.6.5: Maximising yield

- Ensure you keep an accurate academic transcript.
- **Sign up to newsletters** from the surgical colleges and associations, which often contain a wealth of information about bursaries, scholarships and prizes.
- Apply for **many** bursaries / scholarships / prizes; **you only need success with a few** over the years to maximise your scoring.
- **Conferences are excellent opportunities** for point scoring; they show commitment to specialty, facilitate presentation of your work and usually offer many (student) prizes.

> **Common pitfalls**
>
> - Failing to recognise the importance of your academic achievements **relative to your peers**
> - Failing to recognise that an intercalated BSc is **highly regarded in postgraduate applications**
> - **Being unaware** of the available bursaries, scholarships and prizes available and, importantly, the **time of year that you need to apply**
> - **Not giving yourself enough time** to put together applications

6.6.6: Resources

1. Association of Surgeons in Training (ASiT). www.asit.org/resources/grants-awards-bursaries
2. Medical Schools Council (MSC). www.medschools.ac.uk/studying-medicine/medical-student-electives/elective-bursaries
3. Royal College of Surgeons of Edinburgh (RCSEd). www.rcsed.ac.uk/professional-support-development-resources/grants-jobs-and-placements/research-travel-and-award-opportunities/student-bursaries
4. Royal College of Surgeons of England (RCS). www.rcseng.ac.uk/careers-in-surgery/medical-students/prizes-for-medical-students/
5. Royal Society of Medicine (RSM). www.rsm.ac.uk/prizes-and-awards/prizes-for-students/

6.7: Commitment to specialty

> **Golden rules**
>
> Show a **sustained** commitment, by providing evidence of **continued** engagement in relevant activities across the **breadth** of the portfolio themes. The goal is to acquire an **in-depth understanding** of the specialty and to **develop the personal and professional characteristics** needed to excel within it.

6.7.1: Skills demonstrated

Apprenticeship 〉	Leadership 〉〉	Scholarship 〉〉〉
Honest	Committed	Determined
Productive	Conscientious	Motivated
Professional	Disciplined	Organised
Reflective	Interested	
	Self-directed	

6.7.2: Relevance to surgical training

Surgical training is a long and demanding process and so **it is essential that those appointed are insightful and well-equipped enough to complete it.** This is not just important for the trainee, but also the surgical workforce in general. Assessors therefore seek evidence that the decision to apply has come following **careful** consideration of the nature of the training programme, the specialty, and its appropriateness to their character, skill set and expectations.

6.7.3: Getting started

Undergraduate
- Perform well in your exams.
- Undertake your SSCs in anatomy and surgery.
- Join the surgical societies and seek election to their committees.
- Attend courses and conferences in the relevant specialty, looking to present work there.
- Aim to complete and publish at least one research project, QI project and clinical audit.
- Consider an intercalated BSc (in surgery).
- Undertake a surgical elective.
- Maintain a surgical logbook.

Postgraduate
- Appraise your portfolio's weaknesses and address these specifically.
- Undertake surgical FY rotations; this can open doors to publication, QI projects, audits, teaching opportunities and 'getting your face known'.

- Attend surgical courses (e.g. basic surgical skills course, ATLS, CCriSP) and conferences.
- Sit MRCS Part A.

6.7.4: Example opportunities

See the individual sections for domain-specific opportunities.

6.7.5: Maximising yield

- Start early.
- Be interested and enthusiastic.
- Engage in pursuits that address the **full range** of portfolio domains.
- Look for opportunities to **fulfil multiple portfolio domains with a single project**.
- Create a coherent portfolio 'narrative' which demonstrates a clear and developing commitment to the specialty.
- Read specialty-specific 'person specifications' and tailor your portfolio accordingly.
- Keep a record of your pursuits.

Common pitfalls

- **Overcommitting time to *clinical* endeavours**. Although these are of course valuable, they score comparatively low when compared to academic pursuits. Therefore, **ensure your efforts are equally shared** amongst the different portfolio domains.
- **Being excessively focused on a specialty too early** in your training may be detrimental, as it's common to change your preference of specialty. Consider undertaking more general surgical pursuits initially, before becoming increasingly focused as a senior medical student / FY doctor.

6.7.6: Resource

1. Core surgical training person specification (https://specialtytraining.hee.nhs.uk/portals/1/Content/Person%20Specifications/Core%20Surgical%20Training/CORE%20SURGICAL%20TRAINING%20-%20CT1%202021.pdf)

Section 3:

3

The surgical interview

Ch 7: General interview advice 45
    7.1: Preparation 45
    7.2: Interview day 46

Ch 8: Understanding the question 49
    8.1: Closed questions about professional qualities 50
    8.2: Open questions 50
    8.3: Ethics and professionalism 51
    8.4: Clinical scenarios 51
    8.5: Specific knowledge 52

Ch 9: Characteristics assessed at interview – 'buzzwords' 53

Ch 10: Professional qualities 55
    10.1: How to answer questions about professional qualities 55
    10.2: Research 58
    10.3: Teaching and education 61
    10.4: Quality improvement and clinical audit 63
    10.5: Leadership and management 66
    10.6: Communication 69
    10.7: Teamwork 72
    10.8: Working under pressure 75
    10.9: Probity 77
    10.10: Empathy and compassion 79

Ch 11: Open questions 83
    11.1: How to answer open questions 83
    11.2: Why surgery? 85
    11.3: Why this specialty? 87
    11.4: Why this region's programme? 90

11.5: Tell me about yourself...93
11.6: What are your weaknesses? 96

Ch 12: Ethics and professionalism 99
12.1: How to answer ethics and professionalism questions.............99
12.2: Common themes...101
12.3: Practice questions 109

Ch 13: Clinical scenarios 113
13.1: Purpose of this chapter..113
13.2: How to answer clinical questions...114
13.3: General surgery 117
13.4: Trauma and orthopaedic surgery...123
13.5: Vascular and cardiothoracic surgery.....................................130
13.6: Neurosurgery...134
13.7: Plastic surgery 139
13.8: Urology...143
13.9: Ear, nose and throat surgery..146
13.10: Perioperative care...149
13.11: Advanced trauma life support (ATLS) 151
13.12: Managing a theatre list...154

Ch 14: Knowledge-based interview stations 159
14.1: Apprenticeship..159
    14.1.1: Capacity..159
    14.1.2: Consent 163
    14.1.3: Confidentiality 169
    14.1.4: Handover 171
    14.1.5: Triage...173
    14.1.6: Patient safety...175
    14.1.7: Adverse event management 177
    14.1.8: Order of escalation...180
    14.1.9: Challenging consultations 182
14.2: Leadership...184
    14.2.1: Responsibilities in the workplace 184
    14.2.2: Ethical principles...185
14.3: Scholarship...186
    14.3.1: Statistical definitions 186
    14.3.2: Study designs 191
    14.3.3: Patient-reported outcome measures........................196
    14.3.4: Research funding 198

CHAPTER 7:

General interview advice

The way in which interviewees are scored has become increasingly **structured** and so, to facilitate this, marks are awarded for **specific** answers to the **predetermined** questions. The benefit of this system is that training posts should be awarded fairly and meritocratically.

> **Interview tip**
>
> The important consequence of this method of assessing interviewees is that **the surgical 'interview' is now a misnomer; rather, it is a viva** (i.e. an oral assessment/exam). It should therefore be treated like any other exam. The most common mistake made by interviewees is that they do not appreciate the important distinction between an 'interview' and a 'viva'.

7.1: Preparation

7.1.1: Answers

> **Common pitfalls**
>
> You should prepare an answer for every question that is included in this book.

There are very predictable themes of questioning, all of which require a specific type of response, and the details on how to prepare and deliver these are found at the start of every chapter (a summary can also be found in *Chapter 8*). The central requirements for each answer are that it is structured, concise and relevant.

7.1.2: Practising your delivery

Once you have prepared your answers, you must practise delivering them **out loud**: this is essential. Speaking in front of the mirror is usually the best initial method and, once answers are memorised and fluent, practising with colleagues can help to replicate answering under pressure.

The authors have found the following tips to be useful over the years:
- Answer the question specifically.
- Before beginning your answer take a few seconds to recall the key points of your response. This short moment may feel long, but it is time well spent, as it helps to improve the answer's fluency and avoid 'waffle'.
- Speak slowly and clearly.
- Vary your pace and intonation to make answers more interesting to listen to; remember, the interview panel will be repeatedly listening to interviewees all day.
- Deliver your answer with conviction, even if you are not certain it is correct.
- If you do not know the answer to a question, briefly describe (i) how you would find out and (ii) the principles of the answer.

7.2: Interview day

On the day of the interview, it is important to ensure that you're well rested and can avoid stressors. Therefore, ensure that your travel, clothing and interview material is prepared well in advance, and go to bed early.

7.2.1: Attire

Neatly ironed clinic clothes or a suit are advised; it is probably best to avoid any clothing that could divide opinion. Ensure that you're well-groomed and your hair is tidy. Make sure that your shoes are clean.

Whilst these probably sound obvious, you will be surprised by some of the candidates' appearances on the day.

7.2.2: Behaviour

As the surgical 'viva' is not assessing your character in the same way an 'interview' would, you need only display professional behaviours, so don't worry if you feel you're unable to convey your personality in the short time you're with the interviewer. Eye contact, smiling, confidence and courtesy are the most important behaviours to display.

7.2.3: Cue cards

On the morning of the interview, you should practise delivering your answers to the most commonly asked questions – which are likely to come up – as well as revisiting:

- common guidelines
- common treatment algorithms (i.e. ATLS, CCrISP)
- important facts and definitions that you have difficulty memorising.

It may be helpful to write these down on cue cards and take them to the interview with you.

CHAPTER 8:

Understanding the question

The important prerequisites for understanding the interview question, and so constructing a good response, are:

1. **Recognising the type of question being asked**
   It is important you recognise the type of question being asked, as **they have different purposes** and therefore require different responses. The most common question types are described below and include:
   - closed questions about professional qualities (e.g. 'tell me about a time you've demonstrated your leadership qualities')
   - open questions (e.g. 'why surgery?')
   - ethics and professionalism (you're given an ethical or professional dilemma and asked how you would address it)
   - clinical scenarios
   - knowledge-based stations (e.g. 'what is triage?'; 'how do you conduct a prospective cohort study?'; 'what is Gillick competence?').

2. **Delivering the answer in a *structured* way**
   Good interview answers are delivered in a concise and structured manner. In this text, a number of acronyms and aide-memoires are provided to facilitate this (*see below*).

3. **Having the *knowledge and understanding* required**
   As the 'interview' is largely an exam, there will be stations that are purely knowledge-based. In this book, we describe the most common knowledge-based stations and how to answer them.

The questions asked in surgical interviews are reasonably predictable, falling into one of several common question types, described below.

8.1: Closed questions about professional qualities

See *Chapter 10* for more on professional qualities.

8.1.1: Purpose

Describe how you have demonstrated the skill in question and explain why that will make you a better surgical trainee.

8.1.2: Description

These questions are common and tend to reflect the professional characteristics assessed in your application (e.g. leadership, teaching, research) or those central to managing difficult clinical situations (e.g. teamwork, communication, working under pressure).

Answer these questions using the ROSES acronym (see *Section 10.1*).

8.2: Open questions

For more on open questions see *Chapter 11*.

8.2.1: Purpose 1

An opportunity to present your most impressive achievements from a variety of different domains.

8.2.2: Description 1

You can densely pack these answers with achievements from a variety of different domains, such as clinical (which we've termed '*assistantship*'), teaching / training / research / QI / audit ('*scholarship*') and management / leadership ('*leadership*').

8.2.3: Purpose 2

To demonstrate insight into the topic being questioned.

8.2.4: Description 2

These questions tend to be 'why' questions, often about the specialty ('why cardiothoracic surgery?'), location ('why Edinburgh?') or programme ('why run-through?'). This gives you an opportunity to show the examiners that you understand the opportunities and challenges that you're likely to encounter during training.

This type of question can be answered using the OPALS acronym (see *Section 11.1*).

8.3: Ethics and professionalism

For more on ethics and professionalism see *Chapter 12*.

8.3.1: Purpose

To demonstrate that, if faced with challenging ethical or professionalism issues, you maintain patient safety and deal with the issue effectively.

8.3.2: Description

These interview questions are often perceived to be some of the most difficult to answer, as there is no 'correct' answer. Ultimately, this is about demonstrating that you place patient safety first and you can sensitively deal with the issue by being objective rather than accusatory.

The aide-memoire for this type of question is Understand the ISSUE and manage the RISK (see *Section 12.1*).

8.4: Clinical scenarios

For more on clinical scenarios see *Chapter 13*.

8.4.1: Purpose

To systematically evaluate a common clinical scenario, often a surgical emergency, and provide a safe, robust management plan, appropriate to your level of training.

The surgical interview

8.4.2: Description

Clinical topics tend to focus on conditions where there is surgical acuity and are often associated with a common guideline. The trick to answering these well is to be systematic in your assessment and offer a pragmatic management plan, which shows you understand what you 'actually' need to do.

These questions can be answered with the RAPRIOP acronym or using the ATLS / ALS / CCrISP algorithms (see *Section 13.2.2*).

8.5: Specific knowledge

See *Chapter 14* for more on knowledge-based interview stations.

8.5.1: Purpose

To assess your knowledge of 'hot topics' in medicine and surgery.

8.5.2: Description

Interviews often contain knowledge-based stations, and these are challenging as you either know the answer or you don't. Some of the most commonly assessed areas are:

Apprenticeship >	Leadership >>	Scholarship >>>
Capacity	Responsibilities in the workplace	Statistical definitions
Consent		Study designs
Confidentiality	Ethical principles	PROMS
Handover		Research funding
Triage		
Patient safety		
Adverse event management		
Challenging consultations		

All of these topics are described in this book.

CHAPTER 9:
Characteristics assessed at interview – 'buzzwords'

In the table below, the key characteristics of a good surgical candidate are stated; these are usually referred to as 'buzzwords'. They have been categorised by 'apprenticeship', 'leadership' and 'scholarship', although many of these characteristics are applicable to all three domains.

Interview tip
When you're writing your interview answers, it is useful to: • pick 2–3 of these important characteristics • consider how they will relate to your prospective role as a surgical trainee; and • give an answer which *demonstrates* that you have accrued these skills.

Domain	Apprenticeship ❯	Leadership ❯❯	Scholarship ❯❯❯
Description	Relating to your clinical duties	Relating to your leadership and management abilities	Relating to your academic performance, in research, quality improvement and clinical audit
Characteristics	Calm	Articulate	Accountable
	Communicative	Collegiate	Analytical
	Compassionate	Committed	Conflict resolution
	Competent	Conscientious	Decision-making
	Considerate	Critical thinking	Determined

Domain	Apprenticeship ❯	Leadership ❯❯	Scholarship ❯❯❯
	Dependable	Detail-oriented	High standards
	Dexterous	Disciplined	Motivated
	Efficient	Ethical	Negotiable
	Flexible	Innovative	Nurturing
	Honest	Inquisitive	Organised
	Integrity	Intelligent	Patient
	Mentoring	Interested	Reliable
	Personable	Logical	Time managing
	Probity	Moral	
	Productive	Persistent	
	Professional	Resilient	
	Reflective	Self-directed	
	Respectful		
	Self-improving		
	Trustworthy		

Chapter 9: Characteristics assessed at interview – 'buzzwords'

CHAPTER 10:

Professional qualities

10.1: How to answer questions about professional qualities

Questions about professional qualities tend to be very specific, closed questions that will often name the skill they're asking you to talk about. For example:

- *'Describe a time when you've demonstrated leadership.'*
- *'How have you developed yourself as a medical educator?'*
- *'Are you a good team player?'*

The above example questions have a clear purpose; however, some questions may not seem as immediately obvious, although they are still, fundamentally, asking how you have demonstrated the characteristic. Consider the following:

- *'Why do you think some healthcare teams are less effective than others?'*
- *'Is it essential that all doctors have their leadership abilities formally assessed?'*
- *'Do you think undertaking research should be mandatory for surgical trainees?'*

These all appear as if they're asking you to give an opinion, which seems daunting. In fact, all you have to do to answer these well is link them directly back to the pre-prepared, generic answer that you've learnt. Below, we describe an acronym that you can use to help prepare answers for all of the main professional characteristics described in this book.

	Recognise
	Outline
ROSES	Situation
	Events
	Summary

Answers should be around 1.5–2 minutes in length (~250 words)

10.1.1: Before writing your answer

Before you write your answer for each professional quality, consider the following headings and then **utilise them in your answer**.

Candidate experience

Pick an impressive experience that you have on your CV which demonstrates the central professional characteristic being questioned. **Your answer will be based on this**.

Characteristics demonstrated

Pick **2–3 important characteristics** that are essential to being outstanding in the domain being assessed. **We have described these characteristics in the 'Must Mention' tables within each chapter**, so you may wish to consider using these (*see individual chapters*).

Achievements

Pick 2–3 achievements from your CV that you want to include in the answer.

10.1.2: Recognise

Recognise the importance of the professional quality that is being questioned

±

'Bridge' to your answer (if required)

Initially, **'recognise' that the characteristic being questioned is important as a surgical trainee**. This should be brief. For example, if questioned about teamwork:

- *'Teamwork is central to the delivery of excellent healthcare; something that has been demonstrated many times during my time in training and I know will be essential if I am to excel as a surgical trainee.'*

> **Exam tip: How to 'bridge' to an answer**
>
> If the question asked is not explicit about the characteristic they want you to discuss, it is an opportunity for **you** to determine the focus of the question.
>
> For example, using one of the examples from above:
>
> *'Why do you think some healthcare teams are less effective than others?'*
>
> In this instance, you could deliver an answer that focuses on leadership, communication or teamwork. You therefore need to 'bridge' the question to a pre-prepared answer that you'd like to deliver. This is a technique used commonly by spokespeople and is very challenging, so requires practice.
>
> A useful way of bridging is by using the 'ABC' method:
> - **A**cknowledge – similar to 'recognising' the question, you demonstrate that you have heard what is being asked and why it is important
> - **B**ridge – use a phrase that links their question to what you'd like to tell them
> - **C**ontrol – take control of the question and tell the interviewer what you'd like them to hear.
>
> Using the same example:
> - Question: *'Why do you think some healthcare teams are less effective than others?'*
> - Answer: *'The effectiveness of healthcare teams is an essential component of maintaining safe, high-quality care. I think teams vary in their effectiveness due to the presence and absence of some fundamental characteristics of good teamwork; something that has been demonstrated many times during my time in training and I know will be essential if I am to excel as a surgical trainee.'*
>
> As you can see, the question was only briefly specifically addressed, but we have managed to state a number of important points and 'bridged' to begin telling them about our experience working in a team.

10.1.3: Outline

Outline the essential characteristics that are needed to excel in the professional quality.

- *'For me, these are knowing your individual tasks, trusting the ability of others and working towards a shared common goal.'*

10.1.4: Situation

Give a brief description of the situation / experience that you'd like to talk about.

- *'In my capacity as Chair of the university surgical society, I worked diligently to develop these important skills.'*

10.1.5: Events

Give a full description of the situation and the characteristics that you've mentioned in 'outline'.

10.1.6: Summary

Give a punchy summary of the above, reiterating how your abilities in this professional quality will **allow you to excel as a surgical trainee**.

10.2: Research

10.2.1: Research in surgical training

In its publication *Outcomes for Graduates*, the GMC (2020) states that 'newly qualified doctors must be able to apply scientific method and approaches to medical research and integrate these with a range of sources of information used to make decisions for care.' Essentially, you must be proficient in medical research so that you can **make informed decisions about safe, effective patient care**. It is for this reason that research is valued highly in application scoring but, also, that many of the skills developed undertaking research are **directly transferable to surgical training**.

Must Mentions: Essential characteristics for a researcher	
Critical thinking	Academic research requires small details to be given careful attention and, having come to a conclusion, this outcome to be critically appraised. In the high-stakes scenarios that one will encounter in surgical practice this attribute is essential; whether making quick clinical decisions or deciding on treatment options you'll offer patients.
Motivation	Being self-motivated is a core attribute in completing a piece of academic work and an important skill for being successful in surgical training.

Must Mentions: Essential characteristics for a researcher (cont'd)	
Collaborative	The most effective academics collaborate with other authors regularly. As a trainee you will collaborate with other doctors, specialties and allied healthcare professionals.
Understanding data analysis and study design	The ability to critically appraise a study is essential if you are to understand whether its results are relevant to your patients. Proficiency will help you practise evidence-based medicine.
Ethical and safety considerations	All research involving patients undergoes careful scrutiny to ensure it is ethical and safe. Surgical trainees are often involved in recruiting patients to clinical trials and so an understanding of these principles is essential.
Commitment over time	Much like surgical training, academic research is performed over an extended period and demonstrates your ability to commit to something over time.
Data management and protection	This is a core tenet of surgical practice. As a surgical trainee, you will be handling a large volume of sensitive data and it's therefore essential that you understand these principles.

10.2.2: Examples of research

Apprenticeship >	Leadership >>	Scholarship >>>
Academic foundation programme	–	Literature review / Clinical trial / Original study / Case report
–	–	BSc / MSc / MD / PhD

10.2.3: How to answer a research question

Choose one experience, 2–3 'must mention' characteristics and 2–3 achievements from your CV, then use the template:

ROSES

The surgical interview

10.2.4: Example interview answer

Candidate experience
Collected data for a clinical trial, contributed to the data analysis and manuscript preparation.

Characteristics demonstrated
Understanding data analysis and study design; Commitment over time; Motivation.

Achievements
Academic foundation programme; Intercalated BSc; Publication.

Recognise

With the ongoing pursuit to ensure we make the best evidence-based decisions for our patients, proficiency in the language of medical research is becoming increasingly important.

Outline

I think the essential skills needed to achieve this are an understanding of study design, data analysis and remaining committed and motivated over time.

Situation

Having been appointed to a highly competitive post as an academic foundation doctor, I spent 4 months working full-time on a clinical trial and had the opportunity to contribute to writing and submitting the manuscript, which went on to be published in Journal X.

Events

My main responsibility was to perform an initial literature review and, after spending many weeks reviewing abstracts and papers, I've developed an excellent fundamental understanding of the different types of medical research. What I have found especially useful is the ability to critically appraise a research paper; in particular, whether I would have drawn the same conclusions as the authors and, if so, whether I think that the results are relevant to the patients I was working with. These skills were partly developed during my intercalated BSc, but I found utilising those skills in practice an invaluable way of cementing those principles in my learning. Over the 6 months following my academic post, I helped prepare the manuscript with a team of more senior colleagues; they've just invited me back to take part in another project with them.

Summary

In my opinion, there is a need for surgical trainees to have a good grasp of research principles. It's something that I'm really interested in and I believe that the skills I've developed therein will allow me to excel in the training programme.

10.2.5: Synonymous questions

1. Tell me about a time you've been involved in medical research.
2. Do you think surgical trainees should have to undertake research?
3. Have you published any research?
4. Is it important that surgical trainees are research active?
5. Do you think a higher degree is useful for surgical trainees?

10.3: Teaching and education

10.3.1: Teaching and education in surgical training

Developing skill within teaching and education will help you excel in two ways as a surgical trainee; first, your ability to teach juniors and peers, and secondly, your understanding of how you learn. Aptitude in both facets is equally important: you will be central to the delivery of educational activities of your surgical unit and you must know how you learn, so that your training moments are of maximum benefit.

Must Mentions: Essential characteristics for a good medical educator	
Clinical knowledge	Good medical teaching begins with a firm foundation in baseline clinical knowledge
Technical competence	Learners value teachers who are technically competent and recognise the value in teaching technical skills
Supportive	Providing a supportive learning environment, whether that is the physical space or the atmosphere, influences learning
Communication	The ability to communicate effectively facilitates learner interaction with you, meaning students are more likely to answer and ask questions
Enthusiasm	This may be enthusiasm for medicine in general, a specific specialty or delivering teaching

Adapted from Sutkin *et al.*

The surgical interview

10.3.2: Examples of teaching

Apprenticeship ❯	Leadership ❯❯	Scholarship ❯❯❯
Bedside teaching / delivering lectures	Committee membership of an education society	Undertaking educational research
Facilitating on a course	Taking on a formal educational role through the medical school	Formal qualification in education, i.e. PGCME / MSc

10.3.3: How to answer a teaching question

Choose one experience, 2–3 'must mention' characteristics and 2–3 achievements from your CV, then use the template:

ROSES

10.3.4: Example interview answer

Candidate experience
As an FY1/2, they were appointed as a Clinical Tutor and delivered weekly teaching to a group of 6 medical students over 2 years.

Characteristics demonstrated
Clinical knowledge; Supportive; Enthusiasm.

Achievements
Merits and distinctions; Tutor of the Year award.

Recognise
I well remember the contribution that the surgical registrars made to my training – they always appeared to be central to the delivery of teaching within the surgical units and, often, an advertisement for the specialty.

Outline
I think that the key attributes of an excellent medical educator are a deep clinical understanding from first principles, providing a supportive environment for learners and being enthusiastic.

Situation
In my capacity as a Clinical Tutor at the medical school I've worked hard to develop these skills, having been organising and delivering teaching on a weekly basis for the last 2 years.

Events

I've always excelled academically in my training – having gained a number of merits and distinctions in my examinations – which has given me a firm grounding in the basic sciences which underpin surgical practice. This has promoted two characteristics: first, an ability to teach medical students from first principles, which I believe encourages a better understanding and deeper learning and, secondly, a deeper understanding of how I learn, so I can hit the ground running as a surgical trainee. Enthusiasm and the provision of a supportive learning environment I think come hand in hand and, collectively, help the students engage more meaningfully. As the undergraduate medical curriculum becomes increasingly time pressured, I think that these skills in teaching will allow me to continue providing effective, efficient training; indeed, I was awarded 'Tutor of the Year' as an FY1 in recognition of my contribution to undergraduate education.

Summary

As a future surgical trainee, I believe that these skills will allow me to be an asset as an educator within my unit and, as importantly, this role has provided me with an understanding of education which will help me excel as a learner.

10.3.5: Synonymous questions

1. How have you developed as a medical educator?
2. What experiences do you have in teaching?
3. What are the essential characteristics of a good teacher?
4. Why are skills in teaching and education important?
5. How will being a good teacher benefit you as a surgical trainee?

10.4: Quality improvement and clinical audit

10.4.1: Quality improvement and clinical audit in surgical training

Quality improvement (QI) and clinical audit is **essential for delivering safe, effective care** in a modern healthcare setting, where there are increasing resource and population pressures. It is therefore a **core obligation of all surgical trainees**, who are required to complete QI projects and clinical audit in order to progress through their training.

The surgical interview

Must Mentions: Essential characteristics for good QI and clinical audit	
Those of a good researcher	The skills required of a good researcher (see *Section 10.2*) are also needed if one is to be good at QI and clinical audit.
Multidisciplinary	Improving the quality of care involves looking at the broad systems that influence it, which will involve many different teams, rather than just the surgeons.
Patient-centred	QI and clinical audit must be patient-centred, in order to ask pertinent questions, and find resolutions, that will directly influence the quality of care.
Reflective	Many of the best QI projects and clinical audits are as a consequence of reflective practice, where the healthcare provider retrospectively considers how things could have been improved.

10.4.2: Examples of QI and clinical audit

Apprenticeship ❯	Leadership ❯❯	Scholarship ❯❯❯
Completing a closed loop QI project or clinical audit	Leading a medical student through a QI project or clinical audit	Presenting and/or publishing your project
–	Participating in a local / regional / national improvement group	Attending QI and clinical audit courses and conferences
–	–	Completing a QI fellowship

10.4.3: How to answer a research question

Choose one experience, 2–3 'must mention' characteristics and 2–3 achievements from your CV, then use the template:

ROSES

10.4.4: Example interview answer

Candidate experience
Supervised a Year 5 Student Selected Component, helping three students to complete a QI project.

Characteristics demonstrated

Multidisciplinary; Reflective; Considerate of patient safety.

Achievements

Appointed an Honorary Teaching Fellow; Presentation of the work; Awarded a QI prize.

Recognise

It is incumbent upon us, as healthcare providers, to contribute to the continuous improvement in the quality of care that we provide our patients.

Outline

As a doctor who engages in reflective practice, is considerate of patient safety and functions as part of a multidisciplinary team, I believe I'm very well placed to assist in this endeavour.

Situation

Following my appointment as an Honorary Teaching Fellow at the university, I volunteered to supervise three Year 5 medical students undertaking an SSC in quality improvement.

Events

At that time, I had been working in an orthopaedic unit within a small DGH for a few months and had noticed that the FY1 was regularly performing a daily ward round without senior input. Over the following few weeks I liaised with the FYs, the nursing staff and the physiotherapists, many of whom suggested that – although the patients were being seen every day by the Consultant or Registrar – a ward round note was not being documented. As I thought this could possibly represent a patient safety issue, I led a team of 3 medical students in undertaking a closed loop QI project to address this issue.

Over a period of 6 weeks the team performed 3 cycles of change. We presented the work at our regional meeting, as well as at a national QI conference, where we won the 2nd place prize. It was a piece of work of which I'm very proud and this aspect of the unit's practice has significantly improved as a consequence.

Summary

I believe that my qualities in QI and clinical audit will allow me to excel as a surgical trainee, whilst also contributing to the ongoing improvement of safe and effective healthcare.

10.4.5: Synonymous questions

1. Are doctors responsible for helping to improve the quality of care?
2. What do you think are the important qualities of a doctor undertaking clinical audit?
3. Have you presented any QI projects?
4. Should all doctors be active in QI and clinical audit?
5. Do you think surgical trainees are well placed to help with QI?

10.5: Leadership and management

10.5.1: Leadership and management in surgical training

Leadership and management are prominent features of surgical training, far more so than as a Foundation Doctor, and trainees call upon these skills throughout the day. There is an increasing trend towards developing doctors in this role; indeed, *Good Medical Practice* (GMC, 2013) states that 'doctors make an important contribution to the management and leadership of health services'.

See the briefing paper *Doctors' Perspectives on Clinical Leadership*, published by the BMA in 2012 (available at https://www.yumpu.com/en/document/read/18917615/doctors-perspectives-on-clinical-leadership-bma). It provides an insight into the characteristics most valued by doctors in their clinical leaders.

Must Mentions: Essential characteristics for good leadership and management	
Integrity	Good leaders have strong moral principles, which are consistently displayed and uncompromising.
Commitment	Leaders must have belief in their decisions, so that others follow.
Communication	All decisions must be clearly and accurately conveyed to your team, so that they move collectively towards a common goal.
Decision-making	The decisions of the leader have important consequences; it is important that you can make good decisions when called upon.
Accountability	Leaders accept responsibility and, in doing so, impress this upon their team.

Must Mentions: Essential characteristics for good leadership and management (cont'd)	
Delegation	Good leaders recognise the skills of different team members and allocate work to them accordingly.
Empathy	It is important to recognise when a team member is in need and to act accordingly.

10.5.2: Examples of leadership and management

Apprenticeship >	Leadership >>	Scholarship >>>
Ward round / managing junior colleagues	President of a society	Undergraduate teaching
Theatre team	Chairman of a committee	QI and clinical audit

10.5.3: How to answer a leadership question

Choose one experience, 2–3 'must mention' characteristics and 2–3 achievements from your CV, then use the template:

ROSES

10.5.4: Example interview answer

Candidate experience
Led a team of 3 peers in organising a regional conference.

Characteristics demonstrated
Communication; Delegation; Decision-making.

Achievements
Academic FY post; Captain of boat club.

Recognise

Whilst working nights as an Academic FY2 in General Surgery I often assisted in the CEPOD theatre out of hours. It was here that the importance of excellent leadership as a surgical trainee was illustrated, particularly in these emergency cases.

The surgical interview

Outline

I think that the key to being a successful leader in this situation was being a clear communicator, ensuring tasks were appropriately allocated and making decisions in a sensible and timely manner.

Situation

These are skills I had initially fostered during my time as Captain of the boat club, but I believe I've significantly developed these further whilst leading a team in organising a national student conference. Over a 12-month period, I led a team of 3 colleagues and, collectively, we delivered a conference for over 100 medical students and 20 guest speakers.

Events

To aid communication, I organised weekly meetings, set up a team WhatsApp group and delegated tasks both verbally and electronically. This ensured the team were clear on our shared goals and moved forward collectively, which is something I know is important when working as part of a busy surgical firm. Decision-making was also essential; I remember we had a keynote speaker withdraw a week before the conference and, rather than reorganise the schedule to account for this (and so need to redistribute all of this material to delegates), I elected to try to find another, local speaker at short notice. With the help of some of the medical school staff we were able to find another excellent speaker and so avoid potentially disruptive last-minute changes.

Summary

After a year of hard work, I'm proud to say that the team and I effectively organised a very successful conference, which is now running for a third time this year. I believe that these leadership skills I've accrued will allow me to excel as a surgical trainee, who can provide excellent patient-centred care and be a valued member of the surgical team.

10.5.5: Synonymous questions

1. Why is leadership important as a surgical trainee?
2. What do you think are the most important features of a good leader?
3. Have you displayed leadership in your career as a doctor?
4. How do you see your role as a leader and manager whilst training as a surgeon?
5. What is the role of leadership in theatre?

10.6: Communication

10.6.1: Communication in surgical training

Communication skills development is a theme that runs vertically throughout medical school and surgical training. The necessity for effective verbal and written communication **pervades all aspect of surgical practice** and, consequently, it is always assessed as part of the selection process.

Must Mentions: Essential characteristics for good communication	
Completeness	All information that you communicate should be complete, to avoid omissions, oversights and the need for follow-up questions. This is essential as a surgical trainee, where you will routinely be giving clinical advice to more junior doctors.
Conciseness	Concisely conveying information speeds up the communication process. In the time-pressured environment of surgery, this is especially important.
Consideration	When you are conveying information, it is important to be considerate of the receiver's background, such as their level of understanding or education. As a surgical trainee, you will often convey the same message to a number of different people (e.g. the patient, their nurse, the junior doctor and your Consultant), all of which will require you to deliver the information in a different way.
Concreteness	Your communications should be concrete – with a clear, specific message – to reduce the chances of **ambiguity**. As above, this becomes progressively more important as you progress, where you are increasingly called upon to give advice to more junior colleagues.
Courtesy	You should respect the receiver's culture, values and beliefs when communicating information. This is most pertinent when talking to patients.
Clearness	Similar to 'concreteness', clearness reduces the likelihood of a **misunderstanding**.
Correctness	This relates to the correctness of your grammar or syntax, where errors may raise doubts or be seen as careless. This is especially important in your written communication with patients and their families or formal communication with other doctors.

The surgical interview

10.6.2: Examples of communication

Apprenticeship ❯	Leadership ❯❯	Scholarship ❯❯❯
Writing letters (referral, clinical, etc.)	Sitting on surgical committees	Writing a research manuscript
Ward round		Implementing changes from a QI project or clinical audit
Theatre		
Providing clinical advice		

10.6.3: How to answer a communication question

Choose one experience, 2–3 'must mention' characteristics and 2–3 achievements from your CV, then use the template:

ROSES

10.6.4: Example interview answer

Candidate experience

President of the Universities' surgical society.

Characteristics demonstrated

Conciseness; Consideration; Clearness.

Achievements

Organised a surgical seminar series; Secured funding for teaching resources; Awarded a 'medal' at graduation.

Recognise

My experiences within surgery have consistently demonstrated that effective communication is needed pervasively throughout practice, if we are to provide safe and effective care.

Outline

In particular, I think that the need to relay a clear, concise message, whilst remaining considerate of the recipient's level of understanding, is one of the most fundamental characteristics.

Situation

During my tenure as President of the Universities' surgical society, I believe that I have excelled in demonstrating my ability to communicate effectively, and I am particularly proud of how this influenced the committee's success in delivering a series of surgical seminars.

Events

As President, it was my responsibility to chair the meetings of our 15-person team, who were all at various stages of their undergraduate training. In working with such a large team, I found it especially important that my communications were concise, in order to keep our meetings succinct and to the point. This is a skill which I have seen demonstrated regularly by the surgical trainees, often when they are presenting their patients on the post-take ward round. I also found it important to keep my communications clear – especially when we were advertising the seminar series to the student body – in order to avoid chances for misunderstanding. This is a skill that I recognise will become progressively more important as middle-grade, where I will be increasingly called upon to give clinical advice to my juniors. To fund the seminar series, we submitted an application to a medical charity, which required writing a summary for a lay member of the panel. I think that this ability to recognise how the same information may need to be communicated in different ways will be vital as a surgical trainee.

Summary

I am particularly proud of my achievements as part of the surgical committee and, in recognition of my efforts, I was awarded a 'medal' at graduation. I know that these skills I have developed in communication will prove invaluable going forward, if I am to contribute effectively to the delivery of safe and effective patient care.

10.6.5: Synonymous questions

1. What makes an effective communicator?
2. Why is communication important as a surgical trainee?
3. How have you worked to develop your communication skills?
4. Why is effective communication important in theatre?

The surgical interview

10.7: Teamwork

10.7.1: Teamwork in surgical training

Working effectively within a team is a core attribute of a good surgical trainee, who will work in a number of different teams within a single day. Examples include the surgical ward round, operative team, trauma team and on-call team.

Must Mentions: Essential characteristics for good teamwork	
Understand the skills of others	As a surgical trainee, you will have junior doctors working within your team. It's essential that you understand their clinical competencies, so that appropriate tasks can be safely delegated to them, and, conversely, where help or guidance may be needed.
Trust others	Trust is built up slowly over time as teams develop confidence in one another and recognise the unique skills provided by other members. As a surgical trainee, you will work within a team of other doctors and allied healthcare professionals, all of whom contribute to effective, safe patient care.
Recognise your role	Understanding your role and contribution is an essential prerequisite to working effectively within a team.
Share knowledge	Effective and reliable communication processes allow the team to develop a shared understanding. Surgery is a high risk profession and it is essential that, at all times, all team members are on the same page.
Provide a shared common goal	In surgery, this usually relates to the provision of safe and effective patient care. In addition, there are usually many other shared goals throughout the day, such as working to a tight time schedule, ensuring all clinical duties have been fulfilled and that training opportunities are delivered.
Flexibility	In modern healthcare teams the lines between traditional roles are becoming increasingly blurred. Accepting role overlap will help to meet the needs of patients.
Know your tasks	Particularly in high stakes moments, team members must understand their specific roles and tasks.

Must Mentions: Essential characteristics for good teamwork (cont'd)	
Conflict management	Conflict tends to emerge when there is a misunderstanding between team members; a method of effective mediation is therefore required. It is worth noting that, whilst conflict may be destructive, it can also drive creativity and solutions.

10.7.2: Examples of teamwork

Apprenticeship >	Leadership >>	Scholarship >>>
Ward round	Sitting on committees	Writing a manuscript
Theatre		Working on a quality improvement project
On-call work		

10.7.3: How to answer a leadership question

Choose one experience, 2–3 'must mention' characteristics and 2–3 achievements from your CV, then use the template:

ROSES

10.7.4: Example interview answer

Candidate experience
Contributed to the design and delivery of a peer-assisted learning curriculum.

Characteristics demonstrated
Knowing your tasks; Trusting others; Shared common goal.

Achievements
Secured funding for teaching resources; Elected as Chair of a national committee.

Recognise
Whilst on placement in orthopaedics I witnessed the care of a number of major trauma patients, which emphasised the significance of teamwork in surgery; not just within the orthopaedic team, but also between different specialties' teams.

Outline
For me, it highlighted the central importance of a number of teamworking skills in providing effective patient care. Principally, these were knowing the tasks which you

were expected to complete, trusting the ability of others and working collectively toward a shared common goal.

Situation

These are skills I believe I have developed in my role on an education committee at the medical school, where I contributed to the design of a peer-assisted learning curriculum for medical students in their clinical years and helped to secure funding for the educational resources.

Events

I think that the essential prerequisite to our success was developing a shared understanding of what we were trying to achieve from the outset. I found that spending a relatively short period of time at the beginning of the project to ensure our team members were collectively working towards the same goal proved invaluable over the year. This experience also allowed me to understand my personal expectations within the team; the tasks I was supposed to complete, the meetings I was expected to attend, timelines, and so on. I think that uncertainty over responsibilities within a team will only lead to mistakes and, in the context of surgery, I recognise how important it is to avoid this. One skill that I actually found quite challenging – and so I'm very glad I've had an opportunity to develop it – is learning to trust the abilities of the other members of the team. It wasn't easy at first but, as we all got to know each other better and had worked together for a short while, I felt that this trust developed quite naturally. It's actually a characteristic I found especially useful a few years later, when I was elected as Chair of the University medical research society.

Summary

Having spent a lot of time working with surgical teams, the central importance of excellent teamwork has been repeatedly highlighted. As a prospective surgical trainee, I believe that the skills I've developed in my educational role, as well as over many other roles over the years, will allow me to excel as a team player and contribute to the safe and effective delivery of patient care.

10.7.5: Synonymous questions

1. Why are teams within surgery so important?
2. What are some important characteristics of an effective team player?
3. How have you developed your team working skills?
4. Why do you think some healthcare teams are less effective than others?
5. What is the role of effective teamwork in theatre?
6. What are the core skills of a good team player?

10.8: Working under pressure

10.8.1: Working under pressure in surgical training

It is without question that you will encounter scenarios where you are required to make quick, accurate and robust decisions whilst under pressure; indeed, it is so common that you may not realise you're doing so.

In these situations, it is important that you:
- have pre-empted the pressurised situation and made a preliminary plan, in order to minimise its impact
- deal effectively with the situation whilst it is occurring
- reflect on the situation afterwards, to help improve your response to it on the next occasion.

Must Mentions: Essential characteristics for working well under pressure	
Pre-empt and plan	Prior to undertaking a pressurised shift or procedure, think about different components and where stressors are likely to arise. Where possible, make a plan to avoid or offset these.
Prioritise	Have it clear in your own mind on the relative priority of tasks. If something can be safely delayed until another time, do so.
Take a break	It is not possible to continue functioning at a high level if you are not rested; take a break where you can, even if it is only a few minutes every hour.
Work efficiently	Focus on the most important tasks first, remove distractions where possible (not easy...) and delegate appropriate tasks.
Pause	Pausing is an important moment to take in the face of adversity. It is better to pause briefly and consider your next action, so making those actions as effective as possible, rather than automatically responding to a scenario suboptimally.
Perspective	Where a situation becomes overwhelming, try to step back briefly to gain an overarching perspective. Is everything really as critical as you feel it is? Often not.
Ask for help	If you're not sure, ask; if you can't ask, make the safest decision for the patient in that moment.
Reflect	Reflect on how you would do things differently the next time you're faced with the same situation.

The surgical interview

10.8.2: Examples of working under pressure

Apprenticeship >	Leadership >>	Scholarship >>>
On-call shift	Managing the theatre	Presenting your work
Out of hours shifts	Leading an operation	Exams
High risk steps of a procedure		

10.8.3: How to answer a question on working under pressure

Choose one experience, 2–3 'must mention' characteristics and 2–3 achievements from your CV, then use the template:

ROSES

10.8.4: Example interview answer

Candidate experience

Presented a piece of research at an international conference.

Characteristics demonstrated

Pre-empt and plan; Pause; Reflect.

Achievements

International presentation; Research; Commitment to specialty.

Recognise

Working under pressure is a core surgical skill because we, as surgical trainees, are often required to make pressurised decisions, perhaps because the decision itself is life-/limb-saving or, commonly, because of the volume of work we're dealing with at that time.

Outline

Broadly, I think the skills required to mitigate pressure can be divided into pre-emptive planning, pausing before pressurised decisions and reflecting on performance.

Situation

Recently, I delivered a podium presentation of an original piece of research at an international conference.

Events

Whilst I was quietly confident about my ability to present our work, I was anxious about taking questions from the panel and audience afterwards. I therefore made a concerted effort to ensure I was well versed on the seminal papers on the topic, as well as some key recent papers that had been published. Furthermore, I always try to take a few seconds to think about my answer, so allowing me to give a cogent response, rather than responding immediately without thought. Whilst that experience was still stressful, I do think that these two traits allowed me to perform well under pressure. Afterwards, I discussed my performance with my Consultant to ensure that, for future presentations, I'm able to improve my abilities which, in turn, will further ease the pressure of the day.

Summary

Clearly, the ability to work under pressure is essential to flourish as a surgical trainee and, having developed these three skills, I know I have started to develop a firm foundation upon which I can build.

10.8.5: Synonymous questions

1. Describe a time you've had to work well under pressure.
2. Why is coping under pressure important as a surgical trainee?
3. What skills have you developed to help you work well in pressurised situations?
4. How do you think you'll cope in pressurised situations whilst a surgical trainee?

10.9: Probity

10.9.1: Probity in surgical training

The central virtues for acting with probity are demonstrating *honesty, integrity and trustworthiness* in all of your dealings. These are core values of all professionals, but probity is especially important in medicine and surgery where it is essential that **'your conduct justifies your patients' trust in you and the public's trust in the profession'** (GMC, 2013).

Must Mentions: Essential characteristics for demonstrating probity	
Honesty	Honesty is ensuring that you tell the truth at all times, even if things could have gone better.
Integrity	Integrity is ensuring you follow strong moral and ethical principles unwaveringly.
Trustworthiness	Doctors perceived as trustworthy are those in whom patients believe they can place their confidence.

10.9.2: Examples of probity

Apprenticeship >	Leadership >>	Scholarship >>>
Ensuring documentation is accurate and not retrospectively amended	If working privately, your advertisements should be accurate	Your CV
Forms are comprehensively and accurately completed	Your financial dealings	Completing medical reports
You are appropriately informed to be able to consent patients	–	In the reporting of your findings, from research, QI, audit or otherwise

10.9.3: How to answer a probity question

Choose one experience, 2–3 'must mention' characteristics and 2–3 achievements from your CV, then use the template:

ROSES

10.9.4: Example interview answer

Candidate experience
Incorrect antibiotic prescription.

Characteristics demonstrated
Honesty; Integrity; Trustworthiness.

Achievements
Taster week; Incident reporting; Reflective practice.

Recognise

If we – as doctors – are to maintain the trust of patients and the public in our profession, acting with probity is essential in all of our dealings.

Outline

For me, probity is ensuring that I act with integrity, honesty and trustworthiness at all times; not just clinically, but also in my academic and leadership activities.

Situation

As an FY2 I arranged a 'taster week' with a team undertaking complex revision arthroplasty. We were performing a 1st-stage revision for an infected total hip replacement and, postoperatively, I prescribed the antibiotics for the patients. The antibiotic choice had been discussed with the microbiologists at the weekly MDT but, unfortunately, I had misremembered the antibiotic and, consequently, the patient was given a less effective drug for a couple of days before I realised.

Events

Although no lasting harm came to the patient, I felt it was important that I was honest with both the patient and the team about my mistake. I therefore found the Consultant and informed them of the error and, after ensuring that they didn't want to themselves, I also informed the patient. I next completed an 'incident report form' and wrote a reflective entry in my portfolio; ensuring that I learn from these events is important to me, as I don't want to repeat them.

Summary

I think this experience has offered me a valuable insight into how to deal with complications and has demonstrated that, if dealt with honestly and with integrity, you can still maintain trust with the patient. As a future surgeon, I understand that complications are a near certainty and so the lessons from this experience were highly beneficial and have made me a better doctor.

10.9.5: Synonymous questions

1. Tell me about a time you've needed to demonstrate probity.
2. How have you dealt with mistakes in the past?
3. Have you ever made a mistake in your clinical practice?
4. Why is probity important as a surgical trainee?

10.10: Empathy and compassion

10.10.1: Empathy and compassion in surgical training

Empathy is the 'act of correctly **acknowledging the emotional state of another** without experiencing that state oneself' (Markakis *et al.*, 1999), whereas

The surgical interview

compassion – although founded upon empathy – has the additional step of **wanting to alleviate the suffering** that the other person is experiencing (Fernando *et al.*, 2016). As a doctor, these qualities therefore go hand in hand.

Together, these traits foster trust and disclosure within the **patient–doctor relationship,** can be directly therapeutic for the patient and contribute to job satisfaction (GMC, 2016).

Must Mentions: Essential characteristics of empathy and compassion	
Communicating concern	By saying the 'right things' and using body language effectively.
Active listening	Active listening is not just 'hearing' what the patient is saying: it is the ability to demonstrate and maintain interest, avoid interruptions and postpone your evaluation until they've finished speaking.
Patient-centred	The patient should always be at the centre of our clinical decisions which, in turn, influences the quality of the care we provide. Asking yourself 'is this care good enough for my own family?' is a helpful measure.
Emotional attunement	The ability to imagine how another person is feeling and allowing it to resonate with your own emotions.
Willingness to help	A willingness to help others should be an overarching theme in a doctor's practice.

10.10.2: Examples of empathy and compassion

Apprenticeship ❯	Leadership ❯❯	Scholarship ❯❯❯
Dealing with the acutely unwell patient	Your professional relationships with junior colleagues and peers, especially when they are stressed, burnt out, have had a complication, etc.	QI and clinical audit are a reflection of empathy and compassion, whereby you are striving to improve the quality of care
Consenting for an operation	–	–
Breaking bad news	–	–

10.10.3: How to answer an empathy and compassion question

Choose one experience, 2–3 'must mention' characteristics and 2–3 achievements from your CV, then use the template:

ROSES

10.10.4: Example interview answer

Candidate experience

After a sarcoma clinic, providing a 'debrief' session for a medical student.

Characteristics demonstrated

Active listening; Emotional attunement; Willingness to help.

Achievements

A 'thank you' letter from a patient.

Recognise

As a doctor, I believe that there is a requirement to demonstrate these professional characteristics; for me, they are a fundamental pillar of the doctor–patient relationship, fostering trust and disclosure between us, and are therefore essential prerequisites to providing high quality care.

Outline

Empathy and compassion are skills that I've observed in others throughout my training and that I hope to continue nurturing going forward, by ensuring I continue to engage in active listening, demonstrating emotional attunement with my patients and always displaying a willingness to help.

Situation

Whilst working as an FY1, a medical student returned to the ward early afternoon, following a morning sarcoma clinic with the Consultant. They were 'out of sorts' and I wondered if this was due to the events in clinic, where bad news is often broken; this is a situation that I remember very well from my own undergraduate training. On the pretext of asking them to help me review a patient, I took them off the ward and asked if they wanted to 'debrief'.

Events

We ended up walking the corridors of the hospital for about 30 minutes, during which I really just listened to their experience in clinic and tried to understand how it had made them feel. I think it's important to recognise that there are times you simply need to let someone speak without interruption, and I know that this skill will prove useful as a surgical trainee. Afterwards, I let them know that they were welcome to discuss things again if needed, and I hope this willingness to help provided them with some comfort.

Summary

These skills that I have learnt will be valuable as a surgical trainee, during which time I hope to continue providing excellent patient care, which is founded upon the core skill of being able to cultivate a meaningful doctor–patient relationship.

10.10.5: Synonymous questions

1. Describe a time you've demonstrated empathy.
2. Why are empathy and compassion important in surgical practice?
3. What are the characteristics of an empathetic and compassionate doctor?
4. How will demonstrating empathy help you as a surgical trainee?

References

Fernando, A.T., Arroll, B. and Consedine, N.S. (2016) Enhancing compassion in general practice: it's not all about the doctor. *Br J Gen Pract*, **66(648)**: 340–1. doi:10.3399/bjgp16X685741.

General Medical Council (2013) *Good Medical Practice*. Available at: www.gmc-uk.org/ethical-guidance/ethical-guidance-for-doctors/good-medical-practice/domain-4---maintaining-trust

General Medical Council (2016) *Medical Professionalism Matters: report and recommendations*. Available at: www.gmc-uk.org/-/media/documents/mpm-report_pdf-68646225.pdf

General Medical Council (2020) *Outcomes for Graduates*. Available at: www.gmc-uk.org/education/standards-guidance-and-curricula/standards-and-outcomes/outcomes-for-graduates/outcomes-for-graduates

Markakis, K., Frankel, R., Beckman, H. and Suchman, A. (1999) *Teaching empathy: it can be done*. Working paper presented at the Annual Meeting of the Society of General Internal Medicine, San Francisco, CA, April 29 – May 1, 1999.

Sutkin, G., Wagner, E., Harris, I., and Schiffer, R. (2008) What makes a good clinical teacher in medicine? A review of the literature. *Academic Medicine*, **83**: 452–66.

CHAPTER 11:

Open questions

11.1: How to answer open questions

Open questions are an opportunity to present your most important, impressive achievements in an interesting way. They should be engaging, personal accounts that demonstrate your insight into the role you're interviewing for and highlight why you should be appointed.

You must ensure you stay well clear of giving a dull, impersonal narrative review of your CV; the interviewers will have heard many such accounts and you risk blending into obscurity.

You can structure your answer using the following acronym:

OPALS

Outline

Personal

Assistantship
(relating to your clinical duties)

Leadership
(relating to your leadership and management abilities)

Scholarship
(relating to your academic performance in research, QI and clinical audit)

> Memory aid: **'OPALS'** for **OP**en questions'

Where possible, make every component of your answer specific to the programme, location or unit to which you are applying.

Answers should be around 1.5 – 2 minutes in length (~250 words)

11.1.1: Outline

Open with a short, punchy statement that outlines the rest of your answer.

11.1.2: Personal

Making your answer personal will help it to be impactful and memorable; the interviewers are more likely to be actively listening and attentive. Try to think of interesting experiences or anecdotes that have assisted you in making the decision to pursue a career in surgery. Deliver this in an honest and committed way.

11.1.3: Assistantship

Discuss your **clinical and technical** achievements and aspirations here.

The content that you discuss will necessarily vary depending upon the question, but you could consider:
- Achievements – clinical awards (e.g. 'best FY1 in X', 'instructor potential'); surgical logbook; taster weeks; surgical electives and SSCs; outstanding undergraduate exam results; prizes; competence in procedures beyond your stage of training
- Aspirations – work in a centre of excellence in […]; train in a unit with an established track record in […]; opportunity to take on early operative work / independence; work in a supportive unit; opportunities to work in subspecialty areas (e.g. rural medicine, pre-hospital care, major trauma).

11.1.4: Leadership

Discuss your **leadership and management** achievements and aspirations here.

Examples include:
- Achievements – membership of committees and societies; involvement in organising courses, conferences and teaching; leading audit or QI projects
- Aspirations – encouragement to get involved with national projects; in-training opportunities for developing leadership and management experience (i.e. 'chief registrar' posts)

11.1.5: Scholarship

Discuss your **research / QI / audit and teaching / training** achievements and aspirations here.

The scholarship opportunities are often very different between Units. Make sure you thoroughly research the post that you're applying for and the opportunities it can afford. You may wish to discuss:

- Achievements – higher degrees; published and presented research / QI / audit; involvement in clinical trials; designing and delivering teaching; formal training in teaching; changes in practice due to your input; courses and conferences attended
- Aspirations – opportunity for a higher degree; encouragement to be involved with the research efforts of the Unit; culture of research in the Unit; encouragement to attend courses and conferences; culture of teaching and training (i.e. journal clubs, cadaveric sessions, regional teaching).

11.2: Why surgery?

'Why surgery?' is a very common interview question which gives you free rein to demonstrate your distinction. Remember that a competent surgeon is not just clinically proficient; they must also demonstrate excellence in non-technical operative skills, academia, teaching and leadership. This should be reflected in your answer.

Use the table below to jot down your experiences and aspirations to help get started writing your answer.

	Experiences	Aspirations
Assistantship		

	Experiences	Aspirations
Leadership		
Scholarship		

11.2.1: Example answer using OPALS

Outline

Surgery is an exciting and challenging specialty that requires the trainee to possess a broad range of skills, which I have worked hard to develop over the last few years.

Personal

During my elective I had a chance encounter with a Professor of Surgical Education – we started talking in a queue for lunch and, as I expressed an interest in pursuing a surgical career, he invited me along to a seminar later in the day where he discussed the role of resilience in surgery. Alongside being a very inspirational role model, it was also a clear demonstration that the career demands a varied skill mix to excel.

Assistantship

Of course, I do think that surgical excellence begins with an enjoyment of the basic sciences – I remember this being especially obvious during my taster week in orthopaedic surgery – and, having been awarded honours in my medical degree, as well as a 1st in my intercalated BSc, I know I have a firm foundation upon which to build.

During my 4 months as an FY2 in orthopaedics I worked hard to create opportunities to spend time in theatre and I've managed to accrue 50 cases in my eLogbook.

I loved the technical capabilities that operations required, but what I additionally learnt was that an operation isn't simply a 'recipe'; it requires a deep understanding from first principles so that you can safely plan and perform a procedure. For me, the understanding that non-technical skills are essential for the safe delivery of care only deepened my interest and I believe this insight will allow me to excel as a surgical trainee.

Leadership

One of those key non-technical skills is the ability to work well within a surgical team. During my time as Chair of the University Medical Research Society I had the privilege of working within a close-knit team for 2 years. I believe I've developed a number of essential skills in this domain, which I know will help me immeasurably at every stage of training.

Scholarship

I also think that the culture of academia within surgery makes the career attractive. Having undertaken a 1-year period of dedicated research during my BSc and, most recently, completing an Academic Foundation Programme, I hope to undertake a higher degree during my surgical training. We are well placed as clinicians to contribute to the advancement of medical care and I like that a career in surgery encourages that.

Overall, I find the breadth of knowledge and skills that are required to perform well in surgery interesting, and I have worked hard to develop the characteristics during my training so far. I really look forward to my years as a surgical trainee and the inevitable challenges and rewards that this will bring.

11.2.2: Similar questions

1. Why do you want to be a surgeon?
2. What are the characteristics of a good surgical trainee?
3. What is it about surgical training that interests you?
4. What makes an operation successful?
5. Is clinical competence the only important aspect of surgical training?

11.3: Why this specialty?

All surgical specialties are distinct and so have differences that will make them more or less attractive to you. Although your interest in the fundamental knowledge and skill set of that specialty will clearly be important in your

The surgical interview

decision-making, there are a number of other areas of day-to-day practice which you may wish to mention:

- What is the case mix? Is it mainly trauma or elective practice? What are the bread and butter procedures?
- What are the operations like generally? A high volume of short operations or a low volume of long operations? Do they use a lot of specialist instrumentation (e.g. orthopaedics) or is it mainly fundamental surgical skills (e.g. plastic surgery)? Is there an opportunity for training in minimally invasive surgery (e.g. vascular) or robotic surgery (e.g. urology)?
- What are the available subspecialty interests? Is there a culture of hyperspecialisation?
- Until what grade are you resident at night? Is the on-call a middle-grade (e.g. orthopaedics) or senior (e.g. general surgery) led shift?
- Where will you be based? Is the specialty very centralised (e.g. neurosurgery) or will you be working over a large geographical area (e.g. general surgery)?

Use the table below to jot down your experiences and aspirations to help get started writing your answer.

	Experiences	Aspirations
Assistantship		
Leadership		

	Experiences	Aspirations
Scholarship		

11.3.1: Example answer using OPALS

Outline

I think it's important that, in choosing a specialty, one considers all aspects of the career and takes the time to experience the realities of that specialty's practice.

Personal

I undertook two taster weeks in orthopaedics – one in a district general hospital and another in a tertiary-referral centre – where I spent a lot of time with the registrars, trying to understand their daily requirements, and also looking at the consultants' practice. Ultimately, I found that the daily clinical demands and the culture within the specialty are well suited to my personality, skill set and future aspirations.

Assistantship

What struck me about orthopaedic complaints was how disabling and disruptive patients found their injuries; either because a traumatic injury had changed their life in an instant or because they'd struggled for years with a chronic condition. The life-changing, pragmatic solutions offered by orthopaedics really attracts me. Operatively, I enjoyed the challenge of having to understand the biomechanics of the injury and then plan an effective surgical intervention based on first principles – it was much more testing than I was expecting.

I noticed that most of the consultants have a subspecialty interest area for their elective practice but, when on call, are still competent to take on the majority of general trauma. As a keen academic, I like that I will be able to become an expert in a subspecialty whilst also maintaining my skills in trauma, which I think will keep my future practice stimulating.

The surgical interview

Leadership

The majority of the on-call work is undertaken by the middle-grade surgical trainees, meaning that the registrars took on a more managerial role during these shifts. The current registrars said that this freed up time for them to dedicate to training, which I think is a really attractive feature of the specialty.

Scholarship

As the founder of a number of educational resources and having now published two textbooks, teaching is something I draw gratification from and so it is important that I chose a specialty with a rich culture of this. As orthopaedic complaints account for ~25% of all presentations to healthcare it is essential that medical students and junior doctors are well versed in the basics of the specialty; consequently, there has always been a high number of trainees coming through the specialty and I look forward to being actively involved with that in the future.

Orthopaedics is a deeply interesting specialty that makes a meaningful difference. I've taken steps over the years to try to understand the important features of orthopaedic practice and the requirements of trainees. I believe that it is a career that I will find rewarding and interesting, and which will also allow me to follow some of the non-clinical interests that I have developed.

11.3.2: Similar questions

1. Do you know which specialty you'd like to train in?
2. What factors have helped you decide on this specialty?
3. What aspects of this specialty attract you?
4. What is it about your future career that is important to you?
5. Is it only the clinical aspects of this specialty that helped you decide to apply?

11.4: Why this region's programme?

This question is an opportunity to demonstrate your detailed understanding of the region's programme and relate it directly to your personal goals; **not all training programmes offer the same experience**. For example:

1. Apprenticeship:
   - Do you gain experience in all subspecialties? Can you 'personalise' the latter years of training, if desired?
   - Are there many or few hospitals in the region, and are they geographically close or distant? Will you have to move around?

- What formal teaching do they provide?
- What is the culture like? What are the other trainees like?
- Is the unit well-staffed and supported?

2. Leadership:
   - What committees is the region represented on? Is there an opportunity to get involved?

3. Scholarship:
   a) *Research*

   What opportunities are available? Do they have many / few academic surgeons? Is there a culture of undertaking a higher degree? Is there a regular journal club or forum for discussing your academic work?

   b) *Teaching*

   Will you be working with medical students? What opportunities for teaching are available to you?

   c) *Training*

   Does the Unit run courses that you can attend? Are you encouraged to go to international courses? Are you encouraged to go on Fellowship?

   d) *QI and Audit*

   Is there a regular QI and audit meeting? Is there a regular morbidity and mortality (M&M) meeting?

Use the table below to jot down your experiences and aspirations to help get started writing your answer.

	Experiences	Aspirations
Assistantship		

	Experiences	Aspirations
Leadership		
Scholarship		

11.4.1: Example answer using OPALS

Outline

After attending many surgical conferences, I have had the opportunity to chat with surgical trainees from many different programmes across the UK. It has been made quite clear that, although they are similar, different programmes afford different opportunities and have different focuses.

Personal

Having completed an intercalated BSc in oncology, as well as an Academic Foundation Programme, I hope to pursue an academic career and this programme is therefore very well suited to my career aspirations.

Assistantship

This region is one of the few to offer a rotation in orthopaedic oncology, which I find very attractive, as I think this is the subspecialty that I hope to undertake as a Consultant. My understanding is that there is a strong culture for undertaking fellowship training, which aligns well with my future intentions.

As a medical student here, I attended some of the Wednesday morning registrar teaching sessions. I also know that there are monthly education days, as well as an annual mock FRCS, which sound like brilliant resources.

It is quite clear that the clinical expectations and culture on this programme are well suited to my own.

Leadership

As the past President of the University Medical Research Society, I was heavily involved with the organisation of a national conference and it was something that I really enjoyed doing. I understand that there are two large regional conferences held here annually, and so I wonder if there is an opportunity to be involved in their organisation and delivery?

Scholarship

As an aspiring clinical academic, the department's integration with the University is a very attractive feature of this programme; I've read on the website that there is a dedicated 'academic track' and that oncology is one of the research themes of the Unit. Furthermore, there is a very rich tradition of the registrars undertaking higher degrees, so I expect that this pursuit would be well supported as it is part of the Unit's culture.

I have also seen that this department runs an annual international trauma course, with many of the Consultants sitting as part of the faculty. This clearly inspires confidence that the training in this region will be outstanding.

Overall, I have thoughtfully considered my career aspirations and believe that this programme will allow me to flourish as a surgical trainee.

11.4.2: Similar questions

1. What do you know about this region?
2. What aspects of the training programme are important to you?
3. How will this programme allow you to achieve your career aspirations?

11.5: Tell me about yourself

If asked, this question will likely be at the very start of the interview. This is a golden opportunity to **tell the interviewers your most impressive achievements** and, if you answer the question well, there's a good chance that the rest of the interview will be discussing the contents of your response. Spend a bit of time getting the answer to this question right – make it interesting, insightful and personal. Do not fall into the trap of just describing your CV, as they will probably have that in front of them!

The surgical interview

Jot down your experiences and aspirations below to help get started writing your answer.

	Experiences	Aspirations
Assistantship		
Leadership		
Scholarship		

11.5.1: Example answer using OPALS

Outline

Having spent a lot of time with surgical trainees, the impression that I have been left with is that it is a very privileged position; we owe it to our patients and trainers to make the most of this unique opportunity.

Personal

Over the years, I've worked hard to ensure I've equipped myself with the skills needed to hit the ground running on this programme. Perhaps too hard sometimes and so

I'm looking forward to being a little more selective with the opportunities I say 'yes' to in the future!

Assistantship

After achieving a 1st-class honours in my intercalated BSc and honours in my medical degree, I was awarded a number of prizes at graduation, which I think helped me secure a competitive place on an Academic Foundation Programme in central London. As a keen FY2 in orthopaedics I was afforded a number of clinical opportunities in theatre, including performing five DHSs under close supervision, which I've recently reinforced by attending the 'Core Skills in Orthopaedic Surgery' course and the BOTA conference last November. Collectively, my exam performance and clinical experiences have provided me with a very solid foundation in basic orthopaedic sciences.

Leadership

The role of leadership in surgery seemed important when I was on my taster weeks, where I noticed surgeons at different stages of their training taking on increasing responsibility. I think that this staged delegation of increasing responsibility has been mirrored in my CV; I've spent many years working in teams, for example, during my time on the BMA Medical Students Committee, but, most recently, I've led a number of teams on successful projects. These have included my position as Chair of the University Medical Research Society and leading a team to deliver an undergraduate conference; however, what I'm most proud of is how I led a team of 3 authors in writing a textbook, which was published in April.

Scholarship

Lastly, the strong culture of academic research within surgery is something that I'm really attracted to. I've published a couple of papers in peer-reviewed journals and presented their results at a number of international conferences: one of these was awarded 'best oral presentation' at a meeting in the Netherlands. I understand that taking some time out of programme to undertake an MD or PhD is often encouraged and it's an avenue I'd like to explore in more detail.

I believe that my achievements demonstrate that I'm a well-rounded applicant who has strong credentials both clinically and academically. I have developed the skills and attitudes needed to be an outstanding surgical trainee and I hope to be an asset to the Unit in the future.

The surgical interview

11.5.2: Similar questions

1. Take me through your CV.
2. What makes you a good candidate for surgical training?
3. What are some of your most outstanding achievements?
4. What have you done outside your normal clinical responsibilities which helps you stand out from the rest of today's applicants?
5. Are there any weaknesses in your CV?

11.6: What are your weaknesses?

This interview question is notoriously difficult to navigate, with the temptation being to respond with a strength that can masquerade as a weakness – a 'humble-brag'. "*I work too hard*" or "*I'm a perfectionist*" are oft-cited responses and usually come across as disingenuous.

This is an opportunity to demonstrate self-awareness and provide evidence of your willingness and ability to improve in areas that require development. Its purpose is therefore three-fold:

1. Provide **insight** into areas requiring development
2. Demonstrate the **honesty and humility** needed to recognise and admit shortcomings
3. A **growth mindset** and the motivation to address areas requiring attention.

An ability to demonstrate these characteristics is essential for surgical trainees, as you will definitely struggle at different moments throughout your training; this is a certainty. Simply put, you must be able to recognise your weaknesses, as failure to do so means you will fail to progress or, worse, be dangerous with the scalpel.

A quality response can be difficult to construct, but candidates who are able to do so will likely set themselves apart from the rest of the pack.

11.6.1: Approaching the question

Pick one characteristic and one example then use the template:

ROSES

11.6.2: Example interview answer

Candidate experience
Founded a surgical peer-education society

Weakness demonstrated
Task delegation

Achievements
Founded a national teaching programme; Presented at a conference

Recognise

Having spoken at length to current registrars about the requirements of surgical training, and the learning curve that it entails, the ability to acknowledge areas for improvement is clearly an absolute requirement if one is to develop into a safe and capable surgeon.

Outline

One characteristic that I have noticed is especially important is the ability to delegate tasks effectively, and to trust that they'll be completed efficiently and effectively. I saw this being done regularly throughout the day; for example, asking the FYs to chase a scan, asking the nurse to change a dressing, asking that the secretary copy a letter to a colleague, or trusting that the Core Trainee completes the postoperative paperwork. Failure to entrust people with delegated tasks would lead to an unmanageable personal workload, meaning that the surgical trainee cannot focus on more appropriate tasks and learning opportunities.

Situation

This is a skill that I have historically struggled with and I've been told, on more than one occasion, that I can try to 'micro-manage' the team. Recently, having founded a national peer-assisted learning programme, I have endeavoured to improve on this professional characteristic.

Events

In the process of leading on this project, I have been required to increasingly delegate tasks to others, which I've found very difficult. Particularly early on in the project, I felt the need to regularly check in with colleagues, to ensure everything was progressing as planned. However, as I became increasingly familiar with my colleagues – and they too with me – I found it was easier to trust that they had completed their assigned tasks. What I recognised was that in order to feel comfortable delegating an important task, you first need to take the time to learn about the person to whom you're entrusting it. On reflection, I think that this is

The surgical interview

actually a very healthy trait, which will serve me well in working within the surgical team in the near future. Informally, my team members have said I've improved significantly in this area and I hope to continue to do so.

Summary
Overall, I recognise the need to acknowledge areas of weakness as a surgical trainee and I am both self-aware and willing enough to do so. I hope that, as a surgical trainee, this will allow me to excel both clinically and as a colleague.

11.6.3: Similar questions

1. How could you improve as a doctor?
2. Why is it important that surgeons acknowledge their weaknesses?
3. Why is self-awareness important during surgical training?
4. How do you think surgical trainees should respond when they're told they have a specific weakness?

CHAPTER 12:

Ethics and professionalism

12.1: How to answer ethics and professionalism questions

Questions in ethics and professionalism have become a core tenet of surgical interviews; indeed, most interviews will have an entire station dedicated to it. Although there are a broad range of possible questions, the answers generally share many similar components.

You can answer ethics and professionalism questions using the following:

Understand the **ISSUE**

and

Manage the **RISK**

12.1.1: Understand the ISSUE

Information
- Initially, gather as much information as you can about the issue in question. These should be objective **facts, rather than opinion**; you must not rush to conclusions.
- Gather information about the person's **responsibilities that day**. This is of utmost importance from the outset, so that you arrange suitable cover and therefore ensure that patient safety is not jeopardised.

Safety
- Is there an immediate patient **safety risk**?
- Will there be a patient safety risk if the issue is unresolved? This could be either due to the person in question posing a direct risk, or because an essential shift is left uncovered as a consequence of the issue.

Significance
- Try to understand the significance of the issue in question, as this will help you to understand **who needs to be involved**. *Proportionality is absolutely essential* in these questions; is this something that can be dealt with by you alone, or do you need to escalate it?

UrgEncy
- **When must this be addressed by**? Is immediate action needed or can it wait until a more opportune moment?

12.1.2: Manage the RISK

Recommendation and Referral
You have two overall options when managing these issues:
1. Deal with the issue yourself, although you may wish to seek a **recommendation** from someone else, or
2. **Refer** the issue onwards to another person.

Either way, you need to carefully think about the proportionality of your response and so **who you choose to involve is incredibly important** in managing these situations well. The following people are all possibilities (see *Section 14.1.8*, Order of escalation):
- A near-peer
- A senior colleague
- A consultant (yours or theirs)
- A clinical supervisor (yours or theirs)
- An educational supervisor (yours or theirs)
- The Training Programme Director (TPD).

So, the first step in management is deciding *who* you're going to involve, if anyone.

Intervention
What intervention do you think is needed to resolve the issue? This will vary widely depending on the situation; however, there are some general principles you should consider:
- You should generally **speak to the person** in question about the issue *first*.
- The issue should be dealt with at the **lowest possible level of seniority** needed to safely and definitively address it. There will clearly be instances when there is a need to involve senior people from the outset.

- You should generally encourage the person in question to **perform the intervention themselves**. For example, if you think that their Educational Supervisor should know, you should encourage the person in question to tell them (rather than you). If they refuse, or you don't believe they will, then you should do it.
- Always try to address the issue in a **sensitive manner**, **that does not pass judgement and** *saves face*; you do not know why the issue has arisen and the circumstances that surround it. Gossip can be very damaging.

Substitution

If needed, you should take steps to ensure that the **clinical duties of the person are covered** – this is so you ensure there is no risk of affecting patient safety.

- Begin by looking at the rota yourself to see if you can find a reasonable way to get it covered.
- If not, speak to the rota master (in hours) or the managers (out of hours).

Knowledge

It is **essential that you learn** from the ethical and professional issues that arise in the workplace. Consider:

- Personal **reflection** – this is essential, and you may wish to write an entry in your ePortfolio. You can also consider 'debriefing' with a colleague, in confidence.
- Formal methods for learning and improvement – file an **'Incident Report', audit the issue or undertake a quality improvement project** (see *Section 14.1.6*, Patient safety).

12.2: Common themes

Questions on ethics and professionalism tend to be centred around a 'difficult' colleague. The specific question that you're asked on the day is hard to predict, but it will often fit into one of several common themes, which include:

1. **Organising emergency cover for a colleague who:**
   - calls in sick at the last minute
   - doesn't turn up for a shift
2. **Laziness, such as a colleague who:**
   - is consistently late for their shift
   - doesn't complete their work whilst on call

The surgical interview

3. **Intimidation towards you or a colleague, including:**
   - rudeness
   - harassment
   - bullying
   - sexism
4. **Unlawful or dishonest behaviours, such as:**
   - intoxication at work (e.g. drugs or alcohol)
   - falsifying information (e.g. logbook entries, courses attended, qualifications)
   - looking up investigation results inappropriately (their own or a colleague's).

In our experience, these are the sorts of questions that candidates are least confident with, usually because there is no 'correct answer'. However, what is important is that your answer is delivered in a **structured** way, maintains patient **safety** at all times, offers a **proportional** response and that you **learn** from the situation. These are all encompassed by using the aide-memoire (see *Section 12.1*, above):

Understand the **ISSUE**

and

Manage the **RISK**

12.2.1: Organising emergency cover

Understand the ISSUE
Information
- If a colleague calls in sick, or doesn't turn up for work, you should first seek to understand if *they* need assistance (e.g. an ambulance, acute mental health team).
- Next, look at the rota to see what their responsibility that day is; typically, the question is about an on-call shift.

Safety
- Consider whether patient safety is at risk if the shift is left uncovered. The answer will usually be yes, especially if an on-call shift is not covered.

Significance
- Understanding the significance of this problem will allow you to consider who needs to be involved; broadly, rota issues would initially be dealt with by doctors on that rota, then the rota master and, lastly, the hospital managers.

UrgEncy
- Staffing issues are usually urgent and need dealing with immediately, to reduce the chances of compromising patient safety.

Manage the RISK
Recommendation and Referral
- You will generally be capable of dealing with this situation yourself, although you may wish to seek recommendations from your near-peers initially.
- If you are unable to organise cover, urgently contact the rota master (in hours) or the managers (out of hours).

Intervention
- If your colleague is simply running late, you should offer to stay until they arrive (assuming that you are safe to do so).
- If it would be **safe** to leave it uncovered (i.e. a ward shift), other colleagues can pick up the extra work that day.
- If it would be **unsafe** to leave it uncovered (i.e. an out-of-hours shift), the options are:
  - First, speak to your near-peers to see if anyone is willing to cover the out-of-hours shift. This may leave another in-hours shift the following day uncovered, but these are usually easier to sort out.
  - Consider whether you can safely cover the shift. The rules on shift length are confusing but, essentially, you shouldn't work more than 13 consecutive hours.
  - See if any of the senior doctors would be willing to cover the shift at short notice.
  - Once these options are exhausted, you need to contact the rota master (in hours) or hospital managers (out of hours), who can arrange emergency cover. This might be cross-cover of shifts or an emergency locum.

Substitution
- In this question the 'intervention' is 'substitution', so this heading is not applicable.

Knowledge
- Consider undertaking a QI project to look at the rota, to identify if there is scope to improve its robustness.
- Document a personal reflection on the experience in your portfolio.

The surgical interview

> Resource: *'Factsheet – Rota Rules at a Glance'* by NHS Employers
>
> A summary of working hours, including those on call, can be found here: www.nhsemployers.org/-/media/Employers/Documents/ Need-to-know/Factsheet-on-rota-rules-August-2016-v2. pdf?la=en&hash=0DEB8888AFFDF9E9F9CA01CF8D00989A95B89B73

12.2.2: Laziness

Understand the ISSUE

Information

- First, try to understand why your colleague is not completing their work. This may simply be a symptom of other challenges they face, either in their personal life or elsewhere at work. It is exceptionally important in this scenario that you are non-judgemental.

Safety

- Is their laziness causing an immediate patient safety risk? If so, this needs to be addressed first.
- Consider how patient safety might be affected in the long term if your colleague continues to behave in this way.

Significance

- Try to gauge the significance of this issue and therefore who needs to be involved to resolve it. Examples might include:
  - A recent change in behaviour over a few shifts, which you can address yourself or with the aid of near-peers
  - A long-standing behaviour which, despite attempts from near-peers to resolve, continues to be an issue. You will likely be considering escalation at this point.

UrgEncy

- As long as there is no clear immediate threat to patient safety, this sort of issue can be dealt with urgently (rather than immediately), so as to give yourself some time to come up with a thoughtful management plan.

Manage the RISK

Recommendation and Referral

- As described above, recent behavioural changes are best dealt with at a near-peer level, usually by you if possible.

- If the behaviour is long-standing, you might still attempt to deal with it by yourself but recognise that you may need to escalate it if things do not improve.

Intervention

- The first step in resolving this issue is to speak to your colleague about their behaviour. Try to understand if there is anything you can do to help, especially if it is due to difficulties in their personal life (e.g. you could offer to cover their on-call shifts for a while).
- If the person is unwilling to acknowledge the problem and you think it has the possibility of affecting patient safety, you are obliged to escalate this issue:
  o Encourage the person to speak to a trusted senior colleague or their consultant. Advise them that, if they don't, you will have to do so.
  o Remember that proportionality is essential; escalating to their Educational Supervisor or the TPD would be inappropriate at this stage.

Substitution

- Consider if clinical duties need covering and, where possible, organise this.

Knowledge

- Write a reflective essay in your portfolio, exploring what you did well and could have done better in the management of this situation.

12.2.3: Intimidation

Rudeness, harassment, bullying and sexism are often reported in national training surveys and, accordingly, there are now very well publicised campaigns to eradicate these behaviours in surgery. As the perpetrator is often a senior colleague it can make managing these situations very difficult, especially as the consequences may be severe. Nevertheless, it is essential that such behaviours are addressed.

Understand the ISSUE

Information

- Try to remain impartial, rather than accusatory; it might be that there is an innocent explanation for their behaviour.
- Collect objective facts about the behaviour and note them down; it is helpful to have concrete examples of the demonstrated behaviour.
- You may wish to discuss the issue with a **trusted near-peer** to see if they have observed the behaviour, too.

- It is essential that you avoid 'gossip' (as this can result in losing face), so discuss the matter with the fewest people that are required to resolve the issue.

Safety

- Patient safety is not usually of concern in these scenarios.

Significance

- Try to gauge the significance of this issue and therefore who needs to be involved to resolve it. Examples might include:
  - A *recent* behaviour towards:
    - a single person (the most likely scenario at interview)
    - all colleagues (which may represent difficulties in their personal or professional life).
  - A *historic* behaviour towards all colleagues. It is highly likely that this behaviour has been addressed before and, therefore, that there are people already involved in its management.

UrgEncy

- There is no requirement to address these behaviours immediately. Instead, it is best to observe the behaviour over time, to ensure you formulate a thoughtful, robust plan of action.

Manage the RISK

Recommendation and Referral

- Dealing with the issue yourself is preferable, by speaking to the colleague in question directly. However, this is obviously an incredibly difficult situation and, prior to taking this on, it is sensible to **confidentially** seek counsel from a trusted senior colleague or consultant.
- If you feel unable to address it yourself, again seek counsel before escalating the issue. The most appropriate person to escalate to is another Consultant who **works outside the unit**; this is most likely to be your educational supervisor or a previous Consultant from another job.
  - By escalating to someone outside your unit, it permits a more objective assessment of the problem, whilst also avoiding a conflict of interest and gossip.

Intervention

- If you are going to speak to the person directly, it is essential that you are non-accusatory. Simply state the facts and explain how it made you feel. Confidentially document the meeting afterwards.

- If you decide to escalate, ensure you do so as described above.
- You may wish to ask the rota master if they can take you off duties with that person.

Substitution
- Not applicable.

Knowledge
- Write a reflective essay in your portfolio, ensuring that the entry is confidential and the alleged perpetrator is not identifiable from it.

12.2.4: Unlawful or dishonest behaviours

Such activities have the potential to cause patient harm and bring the profession into disrepute. They therefore require immediate, robust action and escalation; these are not scenarios that you should be managing on your own. As there is less subjectivity in the assessment of these actions – when compared to intimidation (*Section 12.2.3*) – the management in these situations is less nuanced.

Understand the ISSUE
Information
- Gather facts on the behaviour as you need to be confident of your allegation.
- If the person is intoxicated, and so cannot work, find out their responsibilities for the day.

Safety
- Generally, these sorts of behaviours will affect patient safety, either directly (e.g. intoxication) or indirectly (e.g. falsifying qualifications or experience, meaning the staff member is not sufficiently trained).
- You therefore have an obligation to address these issues as an emergency.

Significance
- All such activities are highly significant, even if it is considered a single episode. Due to this, escalation will be necessary in almost every scenario.

UrgEncy
- This will depend on the activity. Intoxication requires immediate action, whereas other behaviours may be managed urgently.

The surgical interview

Manage the **RISK**

Recommendation and Referral

- Initially, you should try to deal with the immediate situation, although you may wish to seek counsel from a trusted near-peer for guidance.
- Additionally, you will need to refer this issue on to a more senior colleague.

Intervention

- When you observe these behaviours, you should speak to the person in question directly and inform them of the need to escalate it. Ensure you are objective and non-accusatory.
- Where possible, that person should be advised to escalate it themselves but, failing that, you should inform them that you will be doing so.
  - The most appropriate person to escalate to initially is a consultant **outside the department**; this would usually be their educational supervisor (ES).
  - If you do not know their ES, speak to yours in the first instance.
- At all points, you should aim to save face and avoid gossip, so only involve those who need to know.

Substitution

- Ensure that the clinical duties of the individual are covered. In certain cases, this might be for many months, whilst the issues are being addressed.

Knowledge

- Reflect on your actions; these are very challenging experiences and there is always something to be learnt.

Resource: *'Good Medical Practice – raising and acting on concerns about patient safety'* by the GMC

Guidance for raising and acting on concerns about patient safety can be read here: www.gmc-uk.org/ethical-guidance/ethical-guidance-for-doctors/raising-and-acting-on-concerns/about-this-guidance

The most fundamental point is that 'you have the responsibility to act on it promptly and professionally'.

12.3: Practice questions

As the scope is so vast, you will need to practise answering these types of question repeatedly, using:

Understand the **ISSUE**

and

Manage the **RISK**

1. You've just completed four on-call night shifts working as a CT1 in orthopaedics. The registrar is non-resident at night, and, prior to the start of each shift, they've said "don't wake me; feel free to cope".
2. Every time you have handed over to a colleague, they have been at least 30 minutes late. This has been going on for six months.
3. The ED Registrar passes you in the corridor and asks you who is on call today. They roll their eyes when you inform them who it is and say, "he's rubbish; he never answers the bleep".
4. You and the Registrar have an operating list. At 7:50am the Registrar calls you to say they've woken up hung over, but to just "crack on with the list and I'll be there as soon as I can".
5. You have noticed that one of your colleagues often calls in sick on the days they're supposed to be on a ward-cover shift. On one such occasion, whilst you're on a zero-day post night shift, you bump into your 'sick' colleague in a local coffee shop.
6. You and a colleague have both been granted funding from the study budget to attend a small training course overseas; however, you didn't see them there. When you return, you overhear this colleague telling the TPD that "the course was brilliant".
7. Your night-time colleague does not turn up to take handover at 8pm and they do not answer their phone when called.
8. You overhear one of your fellow CT2s telling a few FY1 doctors that "Tim, the new CT1, is absolutely useless" and that they "shouldn't bother listening to his clinical advice, because it's probably dangerous".
9. A surgical Fellow, who is visiting from Hong Kong, has recently joined your team. Over the last few weeks at least five patients have told you that he is "rude" and "doesn't listen".

The surgical interview

10. You are a male CT1 on your first day in a small unit, where you meet your new CT2 colleague, Sarah. A Consultant walks onto the ward and greets you, before turning to Sarah and saying, "there are only two rules in surgery: firstly, no women and, secondly, absolutely no women".

11. Your Registrar says that they think one of their female colleagues has been increasingly grumpy recently and wonders if they've put on weight.
He decides to look at her medical record on the electronic system and remarks "her beta-hCG is positive".

12. Despite working with a Consultant for four months, they have still not let you perform a single operation; however, your peers often say that this Consultant is "happy to give the knife away".

13. One of the Registrars asks you to complete a Multi-Source Feedback form for them. When doing so, they stay to watch you complete the form and advise you that "everyone just clicks 'excellent' for everything" and insist that you do so. The FY1 on your team confides in you that this also happened to them.

14. One of your fellow CT1s does not look well and has become increasingly dishevelled over the last few months. Your peers think the same thing, with one commenting that they "think he might be living in his car".

15. A surgical colleague casually asks if you would mind quickly taking their blood. You notice that the labels are for a 'bloodborne virus screen'.

16. In the morning meeting you frequently get a 'grilling' from one of the senior Consultants; they don't appear to behave the same way towards your peers. In private, you ask the Consultant why this is, to which they reply, "it's because you don't have a bloody clue about general surgery".

17. One of the FY2s has started their own business providing minor cosmetic procedures, having attended the appropriate courses. On their website they frequently refer to themselves as a 'surgeon'.

18. At the end of the operating list, you and the Registrar are sitting in the office updating your logbooks. They proceed to enter all four cases as 'supervised-trainer scrubbed', but they were not the primary operator at any point that day.

19. One of your CT1 colleagues always finishes their on-call shift on time, despite your other peers often leaving late. You decide to look at the electronic records for patients that they've admitted that day and notice that their entries are identical to the A&E documentation.

20. You are the rota master for the CTs in vascular surgery. At 4:50pm on a Friday you notice that nobody is down on the rota to cover the weekend night shifts.

21. One of the scrub nurses gets uncomfortably close when tying you into your surgical gown. On a few occasions you think you have felt a hand against your back pocket.

22. During the direct lateral approach to the fibula, the Registrar divides the superficial peroneal nerve. They fail to acknowledge this and when you raise it with them, intra-operatively, they say to "just forget about it and don't bother telling the Consultant".

23. One of the patients cared for by your team has had a wound complication post-surgically; this is for conservative management, so they are discharged with early clinic follow-up. A few days later, you start receiving emails from the patient to your NHS email address. The patient's wife is a Charge Nurse on a nearby ward and you wonder if she has given him your email address from the NHS directory.

24. You are in theatre with a Consultant you've not assisted before. Shortly into the second case you drop the Yankauer suction onto the floor, so ask the scrub nurse for a new one. At this point, the Consultant explodes, shouting obscenities at you, and tells you to get out of their theatre.

CHAPTER 13:

Clinical scenarios

13.1: Purpose of this chapter

> **Important**
>
> It is outside the scope of this book to describe the clinical conditions in detail: epidemiology, pathology, anatomy, symptoms, signs, investigations and management are not addressed.

The central purposes of this chapter are to:

1. **Provide robust tools that you can utilise to answer clinical questions at interview.**
   In *Section 13.2* a number of pragmatic tools are provided to assist with:
   - requesting investigations in a logical manner that avoids omissions
   - formulating a robust management for common surgical presentations.

2. **Demonstrate how these tools can be used to answer some common interview questions.**
   The tools are used repeatedly throughout this section, to demonstrate how you can utilise them to structure your answers to commonly asked clinical questions.

3. **State the commonly assessed clinical scenarios within each subspecialty.**
   At the beginning of each subspecialty section, the commonly assessed clinical scenarios and conditions are stated in a table. *It is recommended that you study these in detail,* as it would be very reasonable for them to be assessed at the interview.

   Unfortunately, it is outside the scope of this book to describe them all fully (although, on occasion, some very high yield clinical information is provided).

4. **Reference some of the commonly assessed clinical guidelines.**
    Interviewers should expect prospective trainees to be aware of very commonly
    employed clinical guidelines, and we include a number of these in this chapter.

13.2: How to answer clinical questions

13.2.1: Investigations

It is important that you demonstrate a **thorough, logical approach** to performing
investigations. This will help you provide sensible, robust management plans that
avoid omissions. A template to facilitate this is shown below.

Investigation type	Common tests

Bedside and non-invasive	• Sample specimens that the patient can readily provide:
	  ○ sputum
	  ○ urine
	  ○ stool
	  ○ other fluids (e.g. discharge from surgical wounds or surgical drain output)
	• Ask the nursing staff to perform functional bedside imaging:
	  ○ ECG
	  ○ spirometry

Bloods	1. Arterial or venous **blood gas**: it's useful to consider this first, as it requires a different set of equipment to be taken to the bedside
	  ○ most acute surgical patients will require a measurement of their **lactate**, so this test is usually needed
	
	2. Blood **cultures**: these are generally taken first in the order of draw so, again, it's useful to consider if you need these early
	
	3. 'Routine' bloods including FBC, U&E and LFTs. Do not forget:
	  ○ **coagulation** screen (most surgical patients require this)
	  ○ consider whether your patient needs a **group and save** (G&S) or a **cross-match** (X-match)

Investigation type	Common tests
	4. **Disease- or system-specific blood tests**: there are many examples, which might include uric acid, amylase, lipase, troponin, serum osmolarities, tumour markers (e.g. CA125, CA15-3, CA19-9, CEA), bone profile and others
Non-radiological imaging	• Ultrasound scanning • Echocardiogram
Radiological imaging	• Plain radiographs
Cross-sectional imaging	• CT • MRI
Invasive tests	• Endoscopy • Aspiration (e.g. a joint; pleural effusion; a collection) • Biopsy

> **Top tip: Blood gases and blood cultures**
>
> When considering blood tests, always think of blood gases and blood cultures **first**: they tend to be sent first in clinical practice and it will also help you to avoid forgetting them.

13.2.2: Management plans

The way you structure your management will depend on the type of question you're being asked. These can be broadly categorised into two types:

1. Definitive care of a named diagnosis
2. The acutely unwell patient that requires immediate urgent management.

Definitive care

For these questions it is essential that you don't fall into the trap of giving a brief answer that just states the definitive procedure required. For example, the answer to 'this patient has suspected appendicitis, how would you manage them?' is not 'appendicectomy'! It is essential that you demonstrate a logical approach

The surgical interview

that addresses all of the important steps. This can be achieved by using the following acronym:

RAPRIOP

Reassurance

Reassuring and inspiring confidence in your patient is important. Mentioning this in your answer, albeit **briefly**, demonstrates emotional awareness and helps to frame the rest of your plan.

Advice

This relates to the advice that you give to both the patient and the nursing staff, and examples typically include:

- remain **nil by mouth**
- make them aware of **red flag symptoms** and advise them to inform the nursing staff if they develop
- **provide samples** for testing (e.g. urine / stool)
- mobility and **positioning** (e.g. to remain non-weight-bearing with their leg elevated; to nurse the patient upright; to follow spinal precautions).

Prescription

Prescribe medication (or therapies) that address:

- the **definitive** diagnosis (e.g. an IV heparin infusion for an arterial embolus)
- **symptomatic** management, which should include both **regular and PRN** medications (e.g. analgesia, anti-emetic, laxatives, thromboprophylaxis)

This section also involves the 'prescription' of the **surgical intervention** required.

Referral

Who are you going to let know **within** your team and **outside** your team? The following are commonly contacted, although there are of course many other situation-specific referrals:

- your senior
- the anaesthetists
- critical care
- the theatre coordinator.

Investigations

As per the table at the start of *Section 13.2.1*. This is sometimes not required, if you've already answered it separately.

Observations

It is essential that you inform the nursing staff of the following:

- **frequency** and **type** of observation (e.g. hourly neuro-observations, neurovascular observations)
- to start **monitoring** if needed (e.g. fluid balance, drain output, pressures).

Plan to follow up

When will you return to review the patient again?

The acutely unwell patient

This sort of question is extremely likely to come up at interview. It is an easy opportunity to maximise scoring as the response can almost be delivered verbatim, so **rehearse a stock answer**. Below are some tips for improving your response.

Initially, ensure that you demonstrate to the examiner that you **recognise the acuity** of the clinical scenario:

> *"From the clinical scenario it is clear that this patient is critically unwell and requires immediate intervention."*

Consider whether any **protocols need to be activated** and if any **specific teams** need to be present or informed:

> *"I'd ask the nursing staff to activate the medical emergency protocol via the hospital switchboard and to contact the Consultant's team in charge of this patient's care."*

Management of acutely unwell surgical patients can be done using a number of different protocols including ALS, ATLS and CCrISP. **Identify the one needed and go through it logically**, as per the course instructions (see *Section 13.11*, Advanced trauma life support).

Once the patient has been stabilised, utilise the **RAPRIOP** acronym (*above*) to **formulate a coherent *ongoing* management plan**.

13.3: General surgery

General surgery is the largest specialty and many CTs will therefore complete at least one rotation in it during their training. Questions about general surgical presentations are common in the interview.

Common clinical scenarios include:
* the acute abdomen (see *Section 13.3.1*)
* perforation of the GI tract
* obstruction of the GI tract
* appendicitis
* severe acute pancreatitis (see *Section 13.3.2*)
* postoperative anastomotic leak (see *Section 13.3.3*).

13.3.1: The acute abdomen

Description: severe abdominal symptoms (typically pain), present for ≤5 days, which may indicate life-threatening pathology.

Aetiologies of the acute abdomen

The aetiologies for the acute abdomen can be broadly categorised by organ system, with the most common pathologies being:
* **gastrointestinal:** obstruction (i.e. adhesions, herniae, volvulus, intussusception), perforation, infection (i.e. appendicitis, abscess), inflammatory (i.e. diverticulitis, inflammatory bowel disease)
* **hepatobiliary:** pancreatitis, cholecystitis, ascending cholangitis
* **vascular:** ruptured AAA, mesenteric ischaemia, bowel infarct, colonic ischaemia
* **urological:** pyelonephritis, ureteric colic, testicular torsion
* **gynaecological:** ectopic pregnancy, ovarian torsion, pelvic inflammatory disease
* **respiratory:** basal pneumonia.

You should have a good understanding of the pathophysiology, clinical features, investigation findings and management options for all of these conditions.

There are no British guidelines for the management of the acute abdomen; however, because the differential is so broad and the presentation is often non-specific, the initially work-up is relatively standardised (although it should ideally be tailored to the likely differentials). Pertinent points are highlighted blue in the answer below.

Example answer for the initial management of the acute abdomen
Reassurance
As this clinical presentation may represent a life-threatening pathology, I would reassure the patient that we are going to perform a number of investigations to try to identify the cause as promptly as we can.

Advice

I would request that the nursing staff perform regular observations and ask that they alert the surgical team urgently if the patient deteriorates. If an NG tube or urinary catheter are required, I would ask the nurse to insert these, assuming they are appropriately trained. Lastly, I would instruct the patient to remain nil by mouth whilst awaiting their investigation results.

Prescription

I would ensure that the patient has parenteral analgesia and anti-emetics charted, as well as considering the administration of IV crystalloid or blood products, if indicated.

If there was concern about a perforated viscus or ischaemia, I would prescribe prophylactic antibiotics.

Referral

If the patient was critically unwell, I would make the on-call general surgical registrar aware of the patient; however, if they are stable, I would defer this referral until after the investigation results are available.

Investigations

There are a broad range of investigations that can be useful in the assessment of the acute abdomen and they should ideally be tailored to the clinical presentation. However, where there is diagnostic uncertainty, I would consider requesting:

- *urine specimen for urinalysis and pregnancy testing*
- *stool sample to screen for infection*
- *blood tests to include:*
  - *VBG to look at lactate*
  - *FBC*
  - *renal profile and electrolytes*
  - *liver profile*
  - *CRP*
  - *serum amylase and lipase*
  - *coagulation studies*
- *plain abdominal XR (+ an erect CXR if perforation is suspected).*

Thereafter, a CT abdomen/pelvis with contrast is often a helpful tool and is frequently required.

Observations

The patient requires close observation whilst awaiting the investigation results.

The surgical interview

Plan to follow up

Finally, I would document my clinical assessment *and plan to review the patient when the investigation results are available.*

13.3.2: Acute pancreatitis

Description: an inflammatory condition of the pancreas that, although often only mild, can result in severe, life-threatening disease.

Useful guidelines

1. **World Society of Emergency Surgery (WSES)**
   '2019 WSES guidelines for the management of severe acute pancreatitis'

2. **NICE Guideline 104 (NG104)**
   'Pancreatitis'

Pertinent points are highlighted blue in the answer below.

Example answer for the management of severe acute pancreatitis

Reassurance

Severe acute pancreatitis is a potentially life-threatening condition *with a mortality rate of ~15%; it therefore requires early recognition and management. Patients often feel very unwell and I would therefore reassure the patient that we will be initiating prompt treatment to try to improve their symptoms.*

Advice

I would request that the nursing staff perform regular observations and ask that they alert the surgical team urgently if the patient deteriorates. As patients are often profoundly intravascularly deplete, I would ask the nurse to insert a urinary catheter, assuming they are appropriately trained. Patients do not routinely need to be made nil by mouth.

Prescription

Pain is a prominent feature of acute pancreatitis, so I would ensure that adequate opioid analgesia is prescribed; it is reasonable to consider PCA *(patient-controlled analgesia). It is important to be mindful that* dose adjustment may be required *if organ dysfunction is present.*

Intravenous crystalloid should be prescribed and titrated against the patient's urine output, aiming for a minimum of 0.5ml/kg/hr. I would ensure that PRN anti-emetics are available, as nausea is common.

As I understand it, antibiotics have historically been prophylactically prescribed, but I recognise that this is no longer routine unless there are features of pancreatic abscess or cholangitis.

Referral
As the patient is going to require admission, I would refer this case to the on-call general surgical registrar. Additionally, if the patient looks very unwell, or there is clinical or biochemical evidence of organ failure, I would urgently discuss them with the critical care team.

Investigations
A broad range of investigations are needed for the diagnosis and prognostication of patients with acute severe pancreatitis. I would urgently take a VBG to look at the lactate. FBC, renal profile and a liver profile are required. For diagnosis, a serum amylase and lipase are required; these are usually at least 3x the normal value.

I would request an urgent ultrasound scan to help delineate the aetiology or, if there was diagnostic uncertainty, a CT-AP with contrast is of value.

Observations
I would ask the nursing staff to perform 4-hourly observations and to carefully document the patient's fluid balance, including their urine output and other losses like vomiting.

Plan to follow up
I would calculate the prognostic score, such as the Glasgow–Imrie score or APACHE II, and document this in the notes. My plan would be to review this patient again within the hour, to ensure they are clinically improving.

13.3.3: Anastomotic leak

Description: defined as 'a leak of luminal contents from a surgical join between two hollow viscera' (Peel and Taylor, 1991), an anastomotic leak is a potentially devastating complication of general surgery, where delays in diagnosis and management worsen outcomes. It is therefore a common question in the interview, usually presented as a patient with postoperative abdominal pain.

> **Useful Guidance: ASGBI / ACPGBI Anastomotic Leak Working Group**
> *'Prevention, Diagnosis and Management of Colorectal Anastomotic Leakage'*
>
> This paper is an excellent resource for understanding this common condition. Pertinent points are highlighted blue in the answer below.

Example answer for the management of anastomotic leak

Reassurance

Suffering a postoperative complication is a distressing time for the patient. I would inform them that this represents a spectrum of disease and reassure them that, once the team had a definitive management plan, I would inform them immediately.

Advice

I would make the patient nil by mouth. If there was evidence of ileus or sepsis, I would ask the nurse to insert an NG tube or urinary catheter, respectively, assuming they are appropriately trained.

Prescription

The management of these patients will depend on the severity of their illness. Initially, administration of oxygen, IV fluids and antibiotics is essential, as sepsis is a major contributor to morbidity and mortality.

If the patient is stable, antibiotic treatment alone, with or without percutaneous drainage of any peri-anastomotic collection, may be all that is required. However, if the patient is unstable, or there is evidence of bowel discontinuity, the patient requires surgical intervention to take down the anastomosis, wash out the abdomen and form a stoma.

Referral

I'd refer this patient on to the on-call general surgical registrar and ask for their urgent review. If the patient is haemodynamically unstable, I would also discuss them with the critical care team.

Investigations

I would send a venous blood gas, to assess the lactate, as well as sending blood cultures (prior to antibiotic administration, if practicable). An FBC, renal profile, liver profile, CRP and procalcitonin should also be sent.

If the patient is unstable and the diagnosis is clear, imaging is not routinely required; however, if there is uncertainty and the patient is haemodynamically stable, contrast-enhanced CT scanning is valuable.

Observations

These patients require hourly observations initially. I would ask that the nursing staff also carefully document the patient's fluid balance, to include the output from their NG tube and urinary catheter.

Plan to follow up

I would plan to repeatedly review this patient *over a number of hours, as this is a valuable means of diagnosis when there is any uncertainty.*

13.4: Trauma and orthopaedic surgery

Trauma and orthopaedic surgery is a very common specialty to be assessed in surgical interviews.

> **Orthopaedic Guidelines**
>
> The British Orthopaedic Association Standards for Trauma and Orthopaedics (BOASTs) contain many of the important orthopaedic guidelines.

Common clinical scenarios include:
- compartment syndrome (see *Section 13.4.1*)
- open fracture (see *Section 13.4.2*)
- neurovascular injury (see *Section 13.4.3*)
- septic arthritis (see *Section 13.4.4*)
- cauda equina syndrome (see *Section 13.6.1*)
- necrotising fasciitis (see *Section 13.7.1*)
- assessment and work-up of major trauma (see *Section 13.11*).

13.4.1: Compartment syndrome

Definition: a rise in the interstitial pressure within a closed osteofascial compartment, resulting in compression of the microvasculature.

> **Important Guidance: BOAST**
> *'Diagnosis and Management of Compartment Syndrome of the Limbs'*
>
> This is the definitive guideline for the management of acute compartment syndrome and should be learnt for your interview. The important points are highlighted blue in the answer below.

Example answer for the management of acute compartment syndrome
Reassurance
This is a limb-threatening emergency which requires immediate action, so I would begin by firing a 'warning shot' to the patient, to let them know that we may be going to theatre shortly.

Advice

I would next advise the nursing staff to split all circumferential dressings down to skin, along their entire length, and to raise the limb to level of the heart. If the patient isn't already, I'd also ask for them to be cannulated. I would ask the patient when they had last eaten and taken fluids and, from now, keep them nil by mouth.

Prescription

As compartment syndrome is a painful condition, I would administer a dose of IV opioid and titrate this to their pain. I would prescribe IV crystalloid to ensure the blood pressure remains within normal limits. I think it is also important to ensure that any anticipatory medications are prescribed; in particular, anti-emetics.

The definitive surgical intervention for this patient is fasciotomy so, now that I've taken all immediate interventions, I would take the necessary steps to facilitate this.

Referral

At this juncture there are a number of people that I would like to let know about the patient. Firstly, I'd make the on-call orthopaedic registrar aware and ask them to come and review the patient immediately. I'd also like to call the theatre coordinator to find out what is currently in the emergency theatre and to advise them that this patient needs to come within the hour. Lastly, I'd make the on-call anaesthetist aware of the patient.

Investigations

To ensure the patient gets to theatre in a timely fashion, I'd ensure that all of their bloods were up to date and that they had a valid group and save. It would also be reasonable to send off a creatine kinase and lactate to the laboratory.

I recognise that, if there was clinical uncertainty, monitoring of the intra-compartmental pressure can be utilised, although I am not currently able to perform this procedure.

Observations

N/A.

Plan to follow up

Finally, I would document my clinical assessment and plan to review the patient within 30 minutes.

13.4.2: Open fracture

Definition: any fracture where there is a direct communication with the external environment. You should note that this is often a breach in the skin; however, fractures can be 'internally open' where the fracture opens into the rectum or vagina.

> **Important Guidance: BOAST**
> *'Open Fractures'*
>
> This is the definitive guideline for the management of open fractures and should be learnt for your interview. The important points are highlighted blue in the answer below.

Example answer for the management of open fractures

Reassurance

This is a potentially limb-threatening emergency which requires immediate intervention in the ED. Patients are often distressed by the appearance of the affected limb so I would reassure them that these are common patterns of injury and can be readily treated.

Advice

Having taken the referral, I would ask the ED to call medical photography and administer IV antibiotics, as these should be given within the hour. I'd also find out when the patient last ate and keep them fasted from now, in case they need to go to theatre urgently. Importantly, if the mechanism has been high energy, I would make the patient aware of the 'red flags' for compartment syndrome and ask that they let a staff member know immediately should these develop.

Prescription

I'd ensure that the patient has appropriate analgesia and anticipatory medications, such as anti-emetics, charted. I also think it's important to check that antibiotics have definitely been administered, to avoid it being overlooked.

These patients will require debridement of the wound, the urgency of which varies depending on the wound contamination; if there is marine, agricultural or sewage contamination, this should be performed immediately. This should be performed in the theatre rather than in the ED, unless there are obvious large contaminants that can be easily removed.

Their fracture will require reduction and immobilisation. I would ensure that the wound was dressed with a saline-soaked gauze and covered with an occlusive dressing, once medical photography have seen it. This photograph should be placed in the patient's medical notes.

The surgical interview

Referral
I'd refer the case to the on-call orthopaedic registrar and, if there is a significant soft tissue defect, the on-call plastics registrar, too. It is important that both specialties are involved in the care of these patients.

Investigations
To ensure the patient gets to theatre in a timely fashion, I'd ensure that all of their bloods were up to date and that they had a valid group and save. Radiographs of the fracture and the joints above and below are needed.

Observations
As these injuries typically involve high energy, it is important to remember that they are also at risk of compartment syndrome, so I would ask the nursing staff to commence hourly neurovascular observations of the affected limb. It is also reasonable to consider admitting the patient to an HDU/ITU bed for observation overnight.

Plan to follow up
I would document my clinical assessment and review the patient again if there were any changes in the clinical condition.

13.4.3: Neurovascular injury

Most neurovascular injuries are as a consequence of the orthopaedic injury, so this is what is discussed below. It should be noted, however, that neurovascular injuries may appear as a consequence of orthopaedic intervention (*see box, below*).

> **Important Guidance: BOAST**
> *'Management of Arterial Injuries Associated with Fractures and Dislocations' and 'Peripheral Nerve Injuries'*
>
> You should be aware of the principles of managing these injuries. The important points are highlighted blue in the answer below.

Example answer for the management of neurovascular injury
Reassurance
Neurovascular injury is limb-threatening and requires immediate decision-making. I would therefore explain to the patient that, as soon as a definitive decision has been made, I will update them.

Advice

I would advise the ED to staunch the bleeding, either by applying direct pressure or a tourniquet, and to treat any life-threatening emergencies first; this may be a distracting injury. I would also advise the ED to escalate this injury to the local vascular team. The patient should be kept nil by mouth.

Prescription

Following resuscitation, the traumatised limb should be realigned and splinted, and this will commonly restore the neurovascular supply; however, should the limb remain impaired, urgent surgical exploration is required. This should be performed as a single, joint procedure between the orthopaedic and vascular surgeons, where the blood supply is temporarily restored, followed by skeletal stabilisation and, finally, definitive vascular repair.

Nerves should also be explored intra-operatively and repaired as an emergency; if the team does not have the ability to perform this, the nerve ends should be tacked together with brightly coloured suture material.

Lastly, it is important to consider the risk of compartment syndrome as a consequence of hypoperfusion, so the threshold for performing prophylactic fasciotomies should be low.

Referral

I'd refer this case on to the on-call orthopaedic Consultant and ensure that the vascular registrar has done the same with their senior.

Investigations

It is prudent to ensure that all routine baseline bloods have been taken and, in the context of trauma, these should include a lactate, coagulation screen and a group and save. An ankle-brachial pressure index is of value in the lower limb. Plain radiographs of the injured extremity are required and should include the joint above and below.

Observations

These patients require hourly neurovascular observations, so should be admitted to a ward where the nursing staff are competent in this skill.

Plan to follow up

I would document my clinical assessment and the neurovascular status of the limb. The patient will require regular clinical review, so I would review them hourly initially.

The surgical interview

> ### Special circumstances: Postoperative neurological deficit
>
> Postoperative neurological deficits are common and usually have a benign aetiology; however, if there is a **painful** deficit, this may indicate interposition of the nerve in your surgical fixation or soft tissue repair. It could also be the onset of compartment syndrome. Urgent surgical exploration is warranted in these specific instances.
>
> When assessing a painless postoperative neurologic deficit, consider the following:
> - Did they have **regional anaesthesia**, a block or spinal anaesthetic? It could be that these have just not worn off yet.
> - Was the **patient positioned** in something that could have caused a compressive neuropathy? For example, stirrups are associated with common peroneal palsies.
> - Is the nerve affected near the surgical field? It may have been **stretched in the retractors** intra-operatively.
> - Is the patient in a **tight dressing**? Casts and dressings are a common cause of postoperative neurapraxia and rapidly resolve when the offending item is removed.

13.4.4: Septic arthritis (the hot, swollen joint) in adults

Questions about septic arthritis are usually framed as 'the acutely hot, swollen joint', for which there are many non-surgical diagnoses.

> **Important Guidance: *'BSR and BHPR, BOA, RCGP and BSAC guidelines for the management of the hot swollen joint in adults'***
>
> The work-up of these patients is fairly intuitive, but there are some essential points that you should be aware of. These are highlighted blue in the answer below.

Example answer for the management of the hot, swollen native joint
Reassurance
The hot, swollen native joint requires urgent orthopaedic attention where there is suspicion of septic arthritis, as a delayed diagnosis can result in irreversible articular damage. I'd advise the patient that I will be sending some fluid away to confirm the diagnosis and will update them when we have the results.

Advice

I would ask the referring doctor to send off bloods, including blood cultures, inflammatory markers and serum urate levels. Assuming the patient is not clinically septic, these should be done **prior to** antibiotic administration, as should joint aspiration, so I would ask the ED to hold antibiotic prescription for now. I would keep the patient nil by mouth, pending my review.

Prescription

I'd ensure that the patient has appropriate analgesia prescribed; these should include anti-inflammatories, if the patient is able to tolerate these safely.

Under aseptic conditions in the ED, the most pressing intervention required is joint aspiration, which is typically continued until dryness. I would look at the characteristics of this fluid: is it purulent, turbid, serous, blood-stained or otherwise? This fluid should be sent for urgent microscopy and Gram staining, to identify bacterial infection or crystal arthropathy. It should then be cultured.

If there is a high suspicion of septic arthritis, the patient will require washout of the affected joints so, if I'm able to do so, I would mark and consent the patient and add them to the trauma theatre list.

Referral

Having finished with the patient, I would make my senior aware of their admission.

Investigations

In addition to the investigations I've already discussed, plain radiographs are needed as a baseline image – they are typically normal in acute septic arthritis.

Observations

The patient requires routine clinical observations on the ward, but I would advise the nurse to call me urgently if the observations deteriorate.

Plan to follow up

I would document my clinical assessment and review the patient again only if they deteriorate.

The surgical interview

> **Special circumstances: Prosthetic joint infection** 🔖
>
> It is important to remember that the presentation of septic arthritis in patients with an arthroplasty is sometimes different. Whilst they can present with an acutely swollen hot, red joint, the symptoms are more often indolent and of a lesser severity. Management is largely the same but there are some important nuances regarding joint aspiration: **this is because the consequences of introducing infection into a prosthetic joint are severe**.
>
> Imagine there is a patient with a total knee replacement who presents with pain, mild swelling and erythema overlying their knee. The diagnosis is unclear, so you aspirate their prosthetic joint. In doing so, you inadvertently introduce infection and the diagnosis was actually cellulitis. They are now in a worse clinical position and are going to require revision arthroplasty. It is therefore essential that prosthetic joints are aspirated in completely sterile conditions which, in practice, normally means in theatre.

13.5: Vascular and cardiothoracic surgery

The presentation and management of ruptured abdominal aorto-iliac aneurysms (rAAA) is commonly assessed in surgical interviews.

Common clinical scenarios include:
* Ruptured abdominal aorto-iliac aneurysms (see *Section 13.5.1*)
* Acute limb ischaemia (see *Section 13.5.2*)
* Pseudoaneurysms
* Aortic dissection (see *Section 13.5.3*).

13.5.1: Ruptured abdominal aorto-iliac aneurysms (rAAA)

Definition: haemorrhage through the true wall of the abdominal aorta, with the presence of retro- or intra- peritoneal blood.

> **Guidance: European Society for Vascular Surgery (ESVS)**
> *'Clinical Practice Guidelines on the Management of Abdominal Aorto-iliac Artery Aneurysms'*
>
> This is an excellent guideline for the management of rAAA which, along with NICE guidelines [NG156], should be learnt for your interview. The important points are highlighted blue in the answer below.

Example answer for the management of rAAA

Reassurance

This is a life-threatening emergency which requires immediate surgical management and the patient should be informed that we will shortly be going to theatre.

Advice

If the patient is stable, I would ask that they are taken for an immediate CT angiogram on arrival to the ED; if they are unstable, they should be brought straight to theatre. The patient should be kept nil by mouth and large-bore vascular access gained.

Prescription

Fluid resuscitation should be undertaken, ideally with blood products; however, the target systolic blood pressure is lower at ~70–90mmHg, termed 'permissive hypotension'. Ultimately, the treatment here is surgical repair, either endovascularly or open, and unnecessary interventions should not delay this.

Referral

I would immediately contact the vascular registrar and ask for their urgent review. It is also important to contact the emergency on-call anaesthetist and the theatre coordinator, to ensure the preparedness of the theatre for the patient's arrival.

Investigations

I would ensure that all bloods were sent urgently, and these should include FBC, renal profile, coagulation profile, lactate and a cross-match.

Observations

N/A.

Plan to follow up

I would document my clinical assessment and proceed to theatre, so as to ensure I – along with the rest of the team – am scrubbed in theatre upon the patient's arrival.

13.5.2: Acute limb ischaemia

Definition: an acute (<2 weeks) decrease in arterial perfusion with the potential to threaten the limb.

> **Guidance: European Society for Vascular Surgery (ESVS)**
> *'Clinical Practice Guidelines on the Management of Acute Limb Ischaemia'*
>
> This is an excellent guideline for the management of acute limb ischaemia and should be learnt for your interview. The important points are highlighted blue in the answer below.

Example answer for the management of acute limb ischaemia

Reassurance

This is a limb-threatening emergency which requires immediate action, so I would begin by firing a 'warning shot' to the patient, to let them know that we are going to begin treatment imminently.

Advice

If the patient isn't already, I'd ask for them to be cannulated. I would ask the patient when they had last eaten and taken fluids and, from now, keep them nil by mouth.

Prescription

Intravenous fluids should be prescribed and oxygen administered, to ensure blood pressure and oxygenation remain within normal limits. Analgesia is given to manage pain and any anticipatory medications are prescribed; in particular, anti-emetics.

Intravenous unfractionated heparin is administered and titrated against the APTT, whilst awaiting definitive open revascularisation surgery. This may be thrombo-embolectomy – typically for acute embolic aetiologies – or bypass surgery, for acute-on-chronic occlusions. Residual thrombus may be treated with intra-arterial instillation of thrombolytic agents, such as tissue plasminogen activator.

I would mark and consent the patient for these procedures, if I was appropriately trained.

Referral

At this juncture there are a number of people that I would like to let know about the patient. Firstly, I'd make the on-call vascular registrar aware and ask them to come and review the patient immediately. I'd also like to call the theatre coordinator to find out what is currently in the emergency theatre and to advise them that this patient needs to come immediately. Lastly, I'd make the on-call anaesthetist aware of the patient.

Investigations

The patient requires baseline routine bloods, as well as a creatine kinase *. If readily available, a* CT angiogram *of the lower limb arterial tree should be performed, as long as it would not cause an unacceptable delay to definitive treatment.*

Observations

N/A.

Plan to follow up

Finally, I would document my clinical assessment *and plan to* review the patient within 30 minutes *.*

13.5.3: Acute aortic dissection

Definition: separation of the layers of the vascular wall as a consequence of intramural bleeding within the media, usually due to an intimal tear, leading to a true- and false-lumen.

> **Guidance: European Society of Cardiology (ESC)**
> *'2014 ESC Guidelines on the diagnosis and treatment of aortic diseases'*
>
> The important points of this guidance are highlighted blue in the answer below .

The below answer relates to Stanford type A acute aortic dissection (AAD), which is managed surgically; however, Stanford type B AAD is typically treated medically.

Example answer for the management of type A AAD

Reassurance

Type A acute aortic dissection is a surgically urgent condition *that is associated with a number of important complications. I would therefore assure the patient that all of the imminent investigations are to be expected and are routine, particularly as there is very frequent diagnostic uncertainty in patients presenting with AAD.*

Advice

I would ask that the patient is kept nil by mouth and IV access is obtained. Blood tests, including FBC, renal profile, lactate *, coagulation, group and save,* D-dimer *and* troponins *should be sent expeditiously.* A 12-lead ECG *should also be obtained.*

Prescription

Blood pressure control forms the mainstay of initial medical treatment *, typically with a β-blocker and a vasodilator, such as glyceryl trinitrate.*

Referral
I'd refer this case on to the on-call cardiothoracic registrar and ask for their immediate clinical review and advice.

Investigations
As there is often diagnostic uncertainty, a CXR *is typically performed initially and may demonstrate a widened mediastinum. The most readily available diagnostic test that commonly follows is a* contrast-enhanced CT of the aorta*, which would demonstrate a double lumen.*

Observations
These patients require continuous careful monitoring to identify any complication of AAD *that may arise, including myocardial infarction, cardiac failure, stroke, spinal cord infarct or mesenteric ischaemia.*

Plan to follow up
N/A.

13.6: Neurosurgery

Neurosurgical presentations are extremely common yet, during the early years of medical training, exposure to the specialty is relatively limited and candidates are therefore often intimidated by neurosurgical stations. However, it is important to recognise that neurosurgical care is highly subspecialist and beyond the scope of a CT1/2; decisions are predominantly made by the neurosurgical registrar and critical care.

Therefore, in order to navigate these stations successfully, one simply needs to understand neurosurgical 'red flags', the common investigations and the principles of initial neurosurgical care.

Spinal Surgery Guidelines

Many spinal surgery guidelines are published through NICE. The most pertinent are collated here: https://spinesurgeons.ac.uk/NICE-Guidelines

---

Common clinical scenarios include:
- cauda equina syndrome (see *Section 13.6.1*)
  - other causes of back pain
- head and cervical spine injury (see *Section 13.6.2*)
- spinal injury (see *Section 13.6.3*)
- intracranial bleeds, including EDH, SDH and subarachnoid haemorrhage.

13.6.1: Cauda equina syndrome

Description: compression of the cauda equina leading to bladder, bowel and/or sexual dysfunction. There is not a universally agreed definition, but the commonly accepted features of cauda equina syndrome (CES) include:

- low back pain
- +/– bilateral sciatic nerve radiculopathy
- saddle or genital sensory disturbance
- bladder, bowel or sexual dysfunction.

> **Important Guidance:**
> *Society of British Neurological Surgeons and the British Association of Spine Surgeons*
> *'Standards of Care for Investigation and Management of Cauda Equina Syndrome'*
>
> This is the definitive guideline for the management of CES and should be learnt for your interview. The important points are highlighted blue in the answer below.

Example answer for the management of cauda equina syndrome

Reassurance

Cauda equina syndrome is a disabling surgical condition that requires urgent investigation and management. I would therefore reassure the patient that we will be closely monitoring them, as well as organising urgent imaging.

Advice

I would ask the patient to remain nil by mouth whilst awaiting their scan result. Additionally, I would encourage the patient to empty their bladder, and ask that the nursing staff perform a pre- and post-void bladder scan. This result should be clearly documented in the notes. If there was a very large residual volume, I would ask that the nurse catheterises the patient, assuming they are appropriately trained.

Prescription

The primary aim of initial management is the relief of pain, so I would prescribe opioid analgesia, along with PRN anti-emetics.

Referral

Current guidance suggests that, if there is a high index of suspicion of CES, imaging should be performed prior to discussion with the neurosurgical team; I would therefore await the results of the scan before contacting them. However, I would make my immediate senior aware of the patient, as well as contacting the radiology registrar, to ensure the scan requested is 'vetted' in a timely fashion.

Investigations
I would review the result of the post-void bladder scan to assess the residual volume of urine in the bladder; <100ml is normal and has a high NPV for CES. For diagnosis, an MRI should be performed without delay and should be available 24 hours a day.

Observations
The patient requires routine observation and should be made aware that, if they lose voluntary control of their bladder function, they should make the nursing staff aware immediately, as this indicates progression of the condition.

Plan to follow up
Finally, I would carefully document my clinical assessment and plan to review the patient with the results of the MRI scan.

13.6.2: Head injury

Description: head injury is an exceptionally common presentation and the most common cause of death in people <40 years old.

> **Important Guidance: NICE Clinical Guideline 176 [CG176]**
> *'Head Injury: assessment and early management'*
>
> This is the definitive guideline for the assessment and early management of head and cervical spine injuries. It is a substantial guideline, containing many lists that are commonly assessed in the MRCS exam and at interview. The important points are highlighted blue in the answer below.

Questions on head injury should initially be answered using ATLS principles (see *Section 13.11*, ATLS). Some important aspects of the guidance include:

Reassurance
N/A.

Advice
- If discharging a patient with a head injury, they should be provided with both verbal and written advice.

Prescription
- Manage pain effectively , as failure to do so can raise intracranial pressure.

Referral
- If the GCS is <8, early involvement from *anaesthetics / critical care* is needed to establish a secure airway.
- Refer to neurosurgery if:
  - clinically important finding on the CT head / neck
  - GCS persistently <8
  - deteriorating GCS
  - progressive focal neurological deficit
  - seizure, without full recovery
  - suspected or definite penetrating injury
  - CSF leak
  - confusion persisting >4 hours.
- Emergency transfer to a neurosurgical unit should only be undertaken once the patient is stabilised and other immediately life-threatening injuries have been addressed .

Investigations
- CT scanning is the imaging modality of choice , rather than MRI (*see criteria, below*)
- If the head injury is clinically obvious, ensure it is not a 'distracting' injury; perform a full assessment to look for other clinically important injuries .

Observations
- Admit for observation if:
  - clinically important findings on CT
- If the CT is normal, admit the patient if:
  - GCS has not returned to 15
  - ongoing symptoms, such as vomiting or headache
  - 'other sources of concern'.

Plan to follow up
- Perform serial neurological examination :
  - every hour if low risk
  - within 30 minutes if high risk or the GCS is <15.

The surgical interview

Criteria for performing a CT head in the adult patient (*from NICE CG176*)
Perform a CT head within 1 hour if: • GCS <13 on initial assessment • GCS <15 at 2 hours following the time of injury • suspected open or depressed skull fracture • signs of a basal skull fracture (e.g. haemotympanum, 'panda' eyes, CSF from the ears / nose, Battle's sign) • post-traumatic seizure • focal neurological deficit • >1 episode of vomiting. These criteria are often questioned at interview.

13.6.3: Spinal injury

As with head injury, the assessment and management of spinal injury is standardised and algorithmic.

Important Guidance: NICE Guideline 41 (NG41) *'Spinal Injury: assessment and initial management'*
You should be aware of the principles of managing these injuries. The important points are highlighted blue in the answer below.

Questions on spinal injuries should initially be answered using ATLS principles (see *Section 13.11*, ATLS).

Assessment

High risk features for spinal injury	
Cervical spine ('Canadian C-spine rules')	**Thoracolumbar spine**
• Over 65 years old • Dangerous mechanism of injury (fall from >1 metre or 5 steps, axial load to the head) • Paraesthesia in the upper or lower limbs	• Over 65 years old • Dangerous mechanism of injury (fall from >3 metres, axial load to the head or base of spine) • Pre-existing spinal pathology or osteoporosis • Spinal fracture elsewhere in the column • Abnormal neurology

Spinal immobilisation

Apply full in-line spinal immobilisation for patients with:

- high risk factor on the Canadian C-spine rule
- no high risk factors on the Canadian C-spine rule, but unable to actively rotate their neck 45° to the left or right
- any high risk factor for TL injury.

In-line spinal immobilisation includes:

- placing a rigid collar
- placing head blocks
- placing the patient on a 'spinal scoop' or spinal table
- taping the head to both the blocks and the scoop / table
- remaining supine
- log rolling.

Imaging

Perform a CT if:

- high risk factor on the Canadian C-spine rule
- no high risk factors on the Canadian C-spine rule, but unable to actively rotate their neck 45° to the left or right
- high risk factors for TL injury, associated with *abnormal* neurology
  - N.B. If neurology is normal, but there is a high suspicion of TL injury, a plain radiograph is the 1st-line investigation.

13.7: Plastic surgery

The most likely stations related to plastic surgery are those concerning soft tissue infections or the management of wounds.

Plastic Surgery Guidelines

BAPRAS have published and collated many of the important guidelines, available here: https://www.bapras.org.uk/professionals/clinical-guidance

---

Common clinical scenarios include:

- necrotising fasciitis (see *Section 13.7.1*)
- assessment and management of wounds (see *Section 13.7.2*).

N.B. The assessment and management of burns is a common presentation in plastic surgery practice; however, burns management is highly specialist and unlikely to be assessed at interview.

13.7.1: Necrotising fasciitis

Description: a rare life-threatening necrotising infection of the subcutaneous soft tissue compartments, typically the fascia (although the muscle may be involved). Thereafter, infection can spread rapidly along the superficial and deep fascial planes.

Core knowledge about necrotising fasciitis

Necrotising fasciitis is classified as type I (polymicrobial) or type II (monomicrobial).

The leading symptoms are:
- clinical features of cellulitis with *pain out of proportion to the clinical picture*
- an unwell patient.

On examination:
- Inspection:
  - an erythematous patch with poorly defined margins
  - +/− blistering and bullae
- Palpation:
  - tenderness, extending beyond the margins of erythema
  - woodiness
  - paraesthesia or anaesthesia over the erythematous region
  - +/− crepitus, due to subcutaneous gas formation

Investigations:
- The diagnosis is clinical.
- Calculate the **LRINEC Score** (see www.mdcalc.com/lrinec-score-necrotizing-soft-tissue-infection).
- Bloods → raised lactate, raised glucose, raised WCC, raised CRP, raised urea, raised CK.
- Imaging → not required, but the presence of subcutaneous gas on X/R or CT may raise your suspicion (N.B. the absence of gas has a low negative predictive value).

Management:
- There are no universally accepted guidelines available.
- Emergency surgical debridement of all devitalised tissue is the definitive intervention.
- Antibiotics are given as an adjunct.

The important points are highlighted blue in the answer below.

Example answer for the management of necrotising fasciitis

Reassurance

Necrotising fasciitis is a life- and limb-threatening emergency that requires immediate surgical intervention. I would therefore reassure the patient that we will be addressing this problem quickly and fire a 'warning shot', so that they understand we will need to take them to theatre.

Advice

If not already done, I would ask the nursing staff to obtain vascular access and to send routine bloods, including a blood gas and cultures. If the patient is septic, a catheter should also be inserted and supplemental O$_2$ should be administered. The patient should be made nil by mouth and I would ask when they had last eaten or taken fluids.

Prescription

The most urgent intervention is the administration of IV antibiotics; however, I would also prescribe IV fluids, analgesia and anti-emetics.

Once these initial interventions have been completed, I would prepare this patient for theatre; they require an emergency radical, systematic, 360° debridement of all devitalised tissues, which continues proximally until healthy margins are reached. This is often well beyond the area of cutaneous erythema and will usually require subsequent operations to achieve soft tissue coverage.

Referral

There are a number of colleagues that I would like to contact about this patient. First, the on-call registrars for plastic surgery, anaesthetics and critical care should be asked to review this patient urgently. I would contact the theatre coordinator and place this patient onto the emergency CEPOD theatre list.

Investigations

As necrotising fasciitis is a clinical diagnosis, investigations are not required if there is a high index of suspicion. Nevertheless, a blood gas, blood cultures and routine bloods (including WCC, CRP, urea and CK) are taken. Where there is clinical uncertainty, imaging to look for the presence of subcutaneous gas can be obtained, although gas is not always present.

Observations

Whilst awaiting theatre, the patient requires continuous monitoring of their observations and will therefore need to remain in A&E or be admitted to critical care.

The surgical interview

Plan to follow up

Finally, I would document my clinical assessment *and plan to review the patient within 30 minutes.*

13.7.2: Assessment and management of wounds

Description: the assessment and management of wounds is a common clinical requirement for all levels of surgical trainee. These could be traumatic or postoperative, with or without superadded infection, and the management varies significantly depending on these factors. Consequently, there are no guidelines available.

Clinical advice: Assessment of wounds

If you are asked at interview how you would assess a wound, you may find the following structure helpful.

1. Inspection:
   - Accurately document its **site, shape and size**.
   - Describe its **margins** → regular / irregular
   - Is there soft **tissue loss**?
   - Are there any gross **contaminants**? If so, what?
   - Can you **see the base** of the wound?
   - Are there any evident **traversing neurovascular structures**? Are they intact?
   - Is there **evidence of infection**, such as surrounding erythema or exudate?

2. Palpation:
   - Vascular:
     - Check the CRT and temperature of the distal skin.
     - Palpate the peripheral pulses of any traversing or subtending arteries.
   - Neurological:
     - Sensory: check there is normal sensation in the distribution of any traversing or subtending nerves.
     - Motor: check there is normal sensation in the distribution of any traversing or subtending nerves.

Although the management of wounds varies significantly, there are a number of generic important points, highlighted blue in the answer below.

Example answer for the generic management of wounds
Reassurance

The appearance of wounds can be distressing for patients, so I would reassure them that I will avoid repeated exposures.

Advice

I would ask that the nursing staff accompany me to the consultation, so that they can immediately re-dress the wound afterwards. It is also prudent to contact medical photography, to ensure we keep a record of the wound's progress over time. The patient should be advised to leave the wound dressing undisturbed and informed of the red flags for superadded infection.

Prescription

If I expect that their wound care will cause discomfort, I would ensure that appropriate analgesia and anticipatory medications, such as anti-emetics, were charted, and a PRN dose given prior to the consultation.

I would ask for the nurse's advice on choice of dressing but, broadly, a non-adhesive, occlusive dressing is required. Antibiotics should be given if there is suspected infection.

Referral

It is not possible to provide a generic response for this section.

Investigations

Routine investigations are not often needed, but swabbing exudate is helpful, as are performing routine bloods if there is suspicion of superadded infection.

Observations and Plan to follow up

It is not possible to provide a generic response for this section.

13.8: Urology

Relative to other surgical specialties, urological complaints are generally of lower clinical acuity. This means that urology does not align well with the types of clinical stations that are generally encountered in the surgical interview. It is therefore unlikely, although not impossible, that you will be faced with a urology station.

> **Urology guidelines**
>
> BAUS have published and collated many of the important guidelines, available here: www.baus.org.uk/professionals/sections/academic/guidelines_publications.aspx

Nevertheless, clinical scenarios could include:

- Acute ureteric colic (see *Section 13.8.1*)
  - o this may be presented as the 'acute abdomen' (see *Section 13.3.1*)
- Paraphimosis (see *Section 13.8.2*)
- Testicular torsion (see *Section 13.8.2*)

13.8.1: Acute ureteric colic

Description: an intensely painful condition due to obstruction of the ureter(s), most commonly due to calculi.

> **Guidance: British Association of Urological Surgeons (BAUS)**
> *'BAUS Standards for the Management of Acute Ureteric Colic'*
>
> This is a comprehensive guideline for the management of ureteric colic, which is presented in a clear, digestible format. The important points are highlighted blue in the answer below.

Example answer for the management of acute ureteric colic

Reassurance
Ureteric colic is an exceptionally painful condition and so requires urgent intervention. I would inform the patient that this level of pain is expected, rather than a sign of severe disease, and reassure them that addressing this is the primary aim of our initial management.

Advice
Initially, I would ask that the patient is cannulated and that a urine specimen is obtained. I would instruct the patient to remain nil by mouth, whilst awaiting their test results, and ask that they alert the nursing staff if they develop any 'red flags' for sepsis.

Prescription
Assuming there are no contraindications, NSAIDs should be administered as first-line pain relief, rather than opioids. Due to their possible side-effects, they should be given at the lowest efficacious dose for the shortest possible time needed to improve the patient's pain. PRN anti-emetics are also important.

Emergency surgical intervention is infrequently required for this common condition; however, if the patient is septic, has acutely impaired renal function, bilateral stones, a single functioning kidney or intractable pain, it may be indicated. In these instances, urgent decompression is required, either with a nephrostomy or ureteric stent, under antibiotic cover.

Referral
In such a circumstance, I would contact the on-call urology registrar and ask for their urgent review.

Investigations
The patient will require a number of investigations. First, a urine specimen should be dipped. Bloods including FBC, renal profile, calcium, urate, CRP and a coagulation screen are needed. If the patient was pyrexial, I would also send blood cultures.

The imaging modality of choice is a CT kidney, ureter and bladder (CT-KUB), which should be performed urgently if there is diagnostic uncertainty, a single functioning kidney, or the patient is unwell.

Observations
I would ask that the patient receives 4-hourly baseline observations initially, although this frequency can be reduced if they remain clinically stable.

Plan to follow up
Finally, I would document my clinical assessment and plan to review the patient with the clinical team on the post-take ward round.

13.8.2: Paraphimosis and testicular torsion

Both of these conditions are common referrals to the CT1/2 on-call for urology and you are encouraged to read about these topics in detail. Below, some high-yield points are described:

Paraphimosis	Testicular torsion
• A urological emergency caused by the foreskin becoming retracted behind the glans penis • It is usually iatrogenic • It is a clinical diagnosis • No ischaemia / necrosis → analgesia, penile ring block and manipulation to reduce the foreskin • If there is necrosis or reduction attempts fail → surgical reduction with circumcision (performed as a second, staged procedure)	• A urological emergency caused by twisting of the spermatic cord → ischaemia of the testicle • Most common <25 years old • Diagnosed with ultrasound • Treatment is emergency scrotal exploration within 6 hours • The contralateral testis is also treated during the emergency procedure, to prevent asynchronous torsion of the 'normal' testis

13.9: Ear, nose and throat surgery

Like urology, ENT presentations are difficult to produce 'stations' for at the interview; the common conditions are often either 'medical' (e.g. otitis media, tonsillitis) or catastrophic, so requiring the immediate attention of a senior ENT doctor.

ENT surgery guidelines

ENT UK have published and collated many of the important guidelines, available here: www.entuk.org/guidelines

---

Clinical scenarios might include:
- Epistaxis (see *Section 13.9.1*)
- Deep neck space infections (DNSI) (see *Section 13.9.2*)
- Peritonsillar abscess ('quinsy')
- Post-tonsillectomy bleed

13.9.1: Epistaxis

Description: nosebleeds account for ~30% of all ENT consults and 0.5% of A&E attendances. Clinically, their severity is diverse but, in extreme cases, epistaxis is life-threatening.

Guidance: ENT UK
'Guideline for the Management of Idiopathic Epistaxis in Adults'

There is no universally accepted guideline for the acute management of idiopathic epistaxis in adults; indeed, there are innumerable treatment algorithms readily available, which have often been agreed at a local / departmental level.

A summary of some of the common themes are highlighted blue in the answer below.

Example answer for the management of acute epistaxis
(If catastrophic haemorrhage with haemodynamic instability → use ALS principles.)

Reassurance
Epistaxis is a worrying condition for patients which, furthermore, can be exacerbated by emotional distress. It is therefore important to reassure the patient and attempt to keep them calm.

Advice

Prior to my attendance, I would ask that the nurse ensures the patient is sitting with their head forward, pinching their nares with constant pressure. It can also be helpful to apply ice to the nape of the neck and forehead. The patient should be advised to spit out any blood that runs into their throat, rather than swallowing it, as this is emetogenic.

If appropriately trained, I would also ask that the nurse gains wide-bore venous access.

Prescription

If the bleeding is brisk, tranexamic acid should be administered and any gross coagulopathy should be reversed; however, the mainstay of treatment is procedural, with the specific sequence of interventions often agreed locally.

Broadly, first-line treatment involves direct visualisation of the bleeding vessel, then either cautery or the application of a haemostatic dressing. If this fails, or is not technically possible, nasal packing is required.

Where this has failed, consideration of surgical intervention is required; most commonly, this would be for endoscopic sphenopalatine artery ligation.

Referral

Should bleeding stop readily with first aid measures, the patient need only be referred to a follow-up ENT clinic; however, if they require procedural intervention, it is prudent to refer the case to the on-call ENT registrar for further advice and consideration of admission for a period of observation.

Investigations

In most cases investigations are not needed. However, it is reasonable to take bloods, including an FBC, coagulation screen and group and save.

Observations

These are dependent on the severity of the presentation.

Plan to follow up

This is dependent on the severity of the presentation.

13.9.2: Deep neck space infection

Description: DNSIs are a group of life-threatening infections that affect the deep cervical space of the neck. Their leading symptoms are neck pain and fever, but they will also cause other symptoms – such as airway compromise – depending on their location.

> **Guidance**
>
> These patients are septic and most of the management that you describe will therefore be relating to the treatment of infection. The important points are highlighted blue in the answer below.

Example answer for the management of DNSI

Reassurance

This is a potentially life-threatening condition that requires emergency attention. I would reassure the patient and advise them that a number of investigations and treatments will shortly be commenced.

Advice

I would ask that the nursing staff apply supplemental humidified oxygen and nurse the patient in an upright position. I would also ask that vascular access is obtained and IV antibiotics are administered, if they are appropriately trained. The patient should be made nil by mouth.

Prescription

The initial emergency management is the administration of broad-spectrum IV antibiotics, according to local policy, and IV crystalloid. Saline nebulisers are also of value. Symptomatic treatment with parenteral analgesia and anti-emetics should also be prescribed.

Referral

After initiating the above treatment, I would contact the on-call ENT registrar and ask for their immediate review, as surgical draining of the infection is usually required. Additionally, I would discuss this patient with the critical care team, as they are likely to require a monitored bed.

Investigations

A number of investigations are required, including a blood gas to look at the lactate level, blood cultures, FBC, renal profile, CRP and a coagulation screen.

*If the patient is safe for transfer, a plain radiograph of the cervical spine may show widening of the prevertebral tissues. Cross-sectional imaging with a contrast-enhanced CT scan is diagnostic, but **there is significant risk to the airway**, so an anaesthetic escort is essential.*

Observations
The patient requires continuous observation and should therefore remain in the ED.

Plan to follow up
Finally, I would document my clinical assessment and plan to review the patient again within 30 minutes.

13.10: Perioperative care

These questions are most likely to be about the deteriorating postoperative patient; however, it could be about **any** clinical presentation in the perioperative period. Due to this breadth, it is not possible to comprehensively address these in this book.

Instead, a matrix of common scenarios is presented below, which you should read further about. Practise answering them using the tools provided in *Section 13.2*.

13.10.1: Complications by clinical presentation

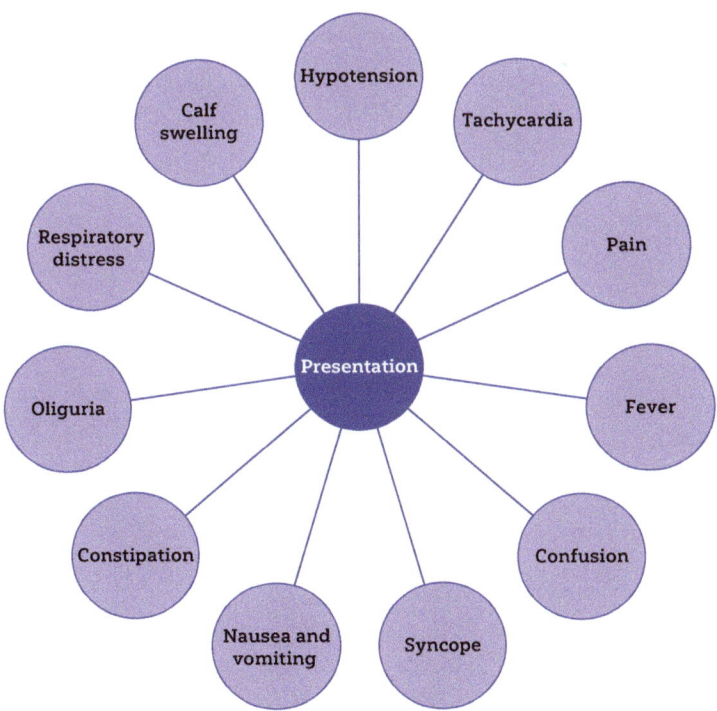

The surgical interview

13.10.2: Complications by pathology

There are some complications that are particular to, or more prevalent within, specific surgical subspecialties, listed below.

Specialty	Complications by pathology
Orthopaedic surgery	• Compartment syndrome (see *Section 13.4.1*) • Neurological injury • Fracture
General surgery	• Anastomotic leak (see *Section 13.3.3*) • Intra-abdominal abscess • Ileus
Neurosurgery	• Raised intracranial pressure • Seizures • Cranial nerve palsies • Intracerebral haemorrhage
Otolaryngology	• Epistaxis (see *Section 13.9.1*) • Cranial nerve palsies • Airway obstruction
Plastic surgery	• Seroma • Haematoma • Threatened flap
Urology	• Ureteric injury • Bladder injury • UTI
Cardiothoracic surgery	• Myocardial infarction (MI) • Stroke • Mediastinitis
Vascular surgery	• Graft failure • Haemorrhage • MI
Non-specific	• Wound dehiscence • Surgical site infection • Venous thromboembolism (DVT and PE) • Lower respiratory tract infection • Neurological injury • Haemorrhage • Cardiac: MI / AF / tachyarrhythmias • Stroke • Metabolic derangements (e.g. hyperkalaemia, hypoglycaemia)

13.10.3: Perioperative clinical information

When presented with this type of question, you may wish to mention a number of pieces of clinical information that you would ascertain prior to reviewing the patient. These include:

- Reviewing the operation note for:
  - any non-standard steps
  - intra-operative complications
  - postoperative instructions
- The indication for the operation
- Type of anaesthesia and regional blocks
- Trends in:
  - baseline observations
  - fluid balance and output (i.e. drains, NG tube, urinary catheter)
  - postoperative analgesic requirements
- DNA-CPR status and ceiling of care
- PMH and DH.

> **Perioperative care guidelines**
>
> NICE have published guidance [NG180] for the general perioperative care of surgical patients. It is available here: www.nice.org.uk/guidance/ng180

13.11: Advanced trauma life support (ATLS)

You should try to attend this course at the earliest possible convenience; it is of high clinical value, assists with answering questions at interview and also scores marks in the application.

ATLS stations are an open goal and there is no reason not to do well. You must simply follow the course instructions systematically, identify the injuries, and commence the immediate life- or limb-saving interventions on a 'see-and-treat' basis. There are two essential prerequisites to performing well in this station:

1. Having a pre-prepared, fluent answer for the primary survey (i.e. 'ABDCE'; this will take up most of the time in the station), and
2. Knowing the general management principles for some of the common traumatic injuries.

The purpose of this section is to demonstrate how to prepare a good answer for the primary survey and to highlight some of the most commonly questioned traumatic injuries, which you may wish to focus more of your attention on.

13.11.1: Primary survey ('ABCDE')

Introduction
This is a high energy mechanism of injury and may therefore represent a multiply-injured patient with immediately life- or limb-threatening problems. I would therefore ensure that the 'enhanced trauma call' is put out, so that the correct members of staff are present on the patient's arrival to resus.

Having taken handover from the pre-hospital team, I would ask the nursing staff to take the patient's baseline observations whilst also commencing my initial assessment and management, focusing on the identification and treatment of life- or limb-threatening conditions.

Airway
I would ensure that the C-spine was triple immobilised with a rigid collar, blocks and tape. Next, I would listen for any noises suggestive of respiratory distress, whilst inspecting the face and neck for any traumatic injuries. I would look in the mouth for vomitus or loose teeth. O_2 at a rate of 15L/min should be applied via a non-rebreather mask.

If prompted, consider:
- jaw thrust (not a 'head-tilt, chin-lift', due to possible C-spine injury)
- airway adjuncts, such as a Guedel or nasopharyngeal airway
- definitive airway – ET tube or surgical (i.e. cricothyroidotomy, if needed).

Breathing
Once the airway was secure, I would move on to assessing their breathing. Initially, I would inspect the chest for evidence of blunt or penetrating trauma and observe for paradoxical respiration. The trachea should be palpated for centrality, as well as the thoracic cage for symmetry of the chest rise. I would percuss the chest for dullness or hyper-resonance and auscultate for breath sounds.

A mobile CXR should be performed.

If prompted, consider:
- emergency needle thoracostomy ('needle decompression')
- surgical chest drain.

Circulation

I would inspect for obvious or occult signs of bleeding, including into the skull, thorax, abdomen, pelvis or externally. The peripheral temperature and capillary refill time should be taken. The rate, rhythm and character of the pulse should be assessed, and the blood pressure taken. A minimum of two large-bore cannulae should be inserted and bloods, including a lactate and cross-match, should be sent urgently. IV fluids should then be administered; this should be O-negative emergency blood if there are concerns of bleeding, otherwise crystalloid is reasonable. Red blood cells, platelets and FFP should be administered at a 1:1:1 ratio, if needed. A cardiac monitor should be applied and a 12-lead ECG taken. I would auscultate the heart sounds.

Next, I would sequentially exam the abdomen, pelvis and long bones for sign of haemorrhage or other injury and request a pelvic XR.

If prompted, consider:
- performing a FAST scan, to look for free fluid
- applying a pelvic binder / ensuring it is correctly located
- applying a tourniquet
- splinting fractures.

Disability

I would ask the nurse to take the patient's temperature and measure the capillary glucose level. I'd assess their pupils for size, equality and responsiveness, and formally calculate their GCS.

Exposure

Lastly, I would fully expose the patient to look for any hidden injuries, and carefully log roll them to assess their spine, back and perineum. If there is suspicion of a pelvic or urethral injury, I would perform a digital rectal examination.

13.11.2: Commonly assessed traumatic injuries

For your clinical practice, you obviously need to learn about the entire breadth of traumatic injuries, as described in the ATLS course manual. Anecdotally, our experience is that the following conditions often come up in the interview:

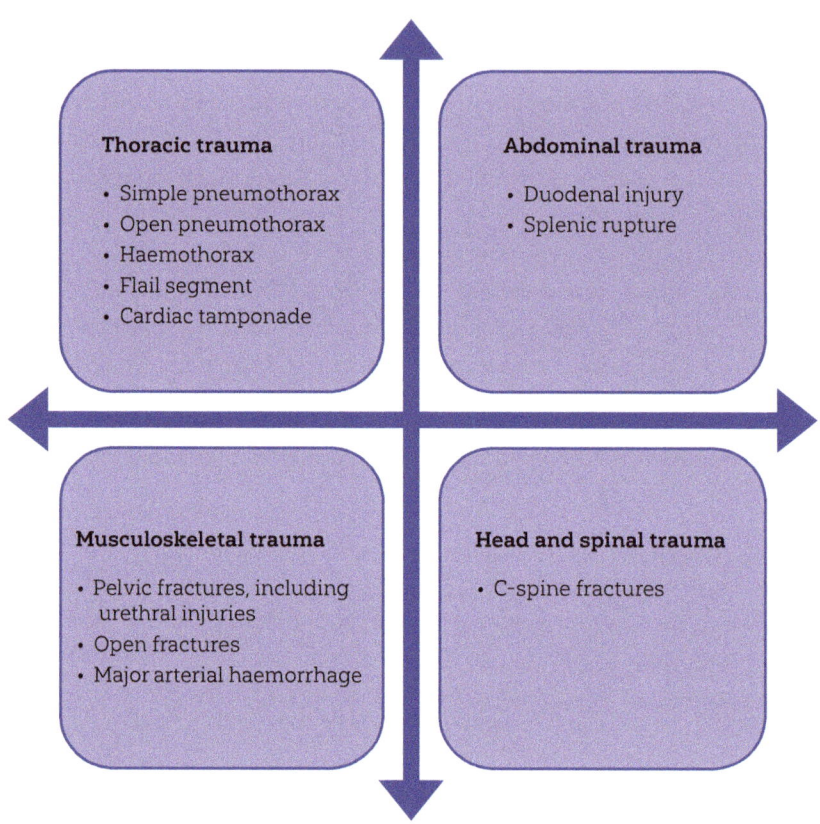

Thoracic trauma

- Simple pneumothorax
- Open pneumothorax
- Haemothorax
- Flail segment
- Cardiac tamponade

Abdominal trauma

- Duodenal injury
- Splenic rupture

Musculoskeletal trauma

- Pelvic fractures, including urethral injuries
- Open fractures
- Major arterial haemorrhage

Head and spinal trauma

- C-spine fractures

13.12: Managing a theatre list

Managing a theatre list is a complex surgical skill, usually done in discussion with the Consultant in charge of the list. Still, clinical scenarios regarding the management of an operating list are common. They tend to refer to either:

- selecting the order for the **next day's** urgent operating list within a specialty,

or

- managing an **emergency** operating list (e.g. multiple specialties contending for priority in the emergency theatre).

There are many principles that should be considered when ordering the list (below). We are aiming to run a theatre that **prioritises patients based on clinical need** and is **safe, effective and time-efficient.**

13.12.1: Patient factors

- With what **clinical urgency** do they need to go to theatre? This is categorised using the NCEPOD Classification of Intervention into immediate, urgent, expedited and elective (see *Section 14.1.5* for a complete description).
- Are there factors which mean the patient should go **early** on the list?
  - **Diabetes mellitus** – these patients should miss as few meals as possible, as poor glycaemic control in the perioperative period increases mortality and morbidity (such as infection, cerebrovascular accident (CVA), MI, pressure sores, others).
  - **Severe allergy** – particularly to latex or iodine, as these are commonly used in theatre. These patients should ideally be first on the list and all offending items in the theatre should be removed, to avoid accidental contact.
  - **Clinically deteriorating patients or very comorbid patients** – these patient groups require senior staff availability and may need a HDU / ITU bed, so should be done earlier in the day.
  - **Time-critical conditions** – is there a time limit within which it is essential that the procedure is performed? Is there national guidance about theatre timing that we should be aiming for?
  - **In the absence of any compelling clinical reason to place a patient first, it is usually best to start the list with a simple case** (from both a surgical, anaesthetic and kit perspective) as this will allow the theatre to get up and running in a timely fashion.
- Are there factors which mean the patient should go **last** on the theatre list?
  - **Infectious cases** – assuming the patient is clinically stable, infectious cases (e.g. MRSA or VRE) should be done last on the list as the theatre will need a deep clean afterwards. If these cases are done elsewhere on the list, there will be an unavoidable delay whilst the theatre is being prepared for the following patient.
- Is the patient medically optimised and have they had all pre-operative checks completed? **Where there is uncertainty or checks haven't been completed, the patient should *not* be first** (unless clinically necessary) as this will delay the theatre and may lead to cancellations.

13.12.2: Staffing and theatre factors

- The **expertise** of the available surgeons, anaesthetists and theatre staff:
  - ○ **Surgeons** – what grade is the surgeon? What is their scope of practice? Do they have a subspecialty practice? Cases should be allocated on these bases.
  - ○ **Anaesthetist** – similar to the above. Some procedures require very specialist anaesthetic skills, such as paediatrics, transplant, cardiothoracic and neurosurgery.
  - ○ **Theatre staff** – are the theatre staff appropriately trained using the kit that is required for the operation?
- **Equipment and tray availability**, including access to appropriate **imaging**.
- **Availability of other subspecialties** – some patients may be best treated with a single procedure during which multiple specialties are present (e.g. open fractures with orthopaedics and plastics in theatre). What time is the other specialty available?
- **Available theatres** – is there any capacity on other theatres, such as the elective lists, the emergency ('CEPOD') theatre or other specialties' lists?

Reference

Peel, A.L. and Taylor, E.W. (1991) Proposed definitions for the audit of postoperative infection: a discussion paper. Surgical Infection Study Group. *Ann R Coll Surg Engl*, **73(6):** 385–8.

What should you do if there is no capacity to take your emergency case to theatre?

You may be faced with this scenario occasionally and it's important that you know what do to. Consequently, this is a common interview question. Your order of escalation should be as follows:

1. The first question is 'is there an **absolute** requirement to take this patient to theatre *now*?'. The NCEPOD states that non-emergency cases should not be performed out-of-hours unless absolutely necessary; so, **could it be safely delayed** until the next available theatre slot on an urgent list?

   No

2. Can any of the other cases currently on the *emergency* theatre list be delayed **safely**?

   No

3. Can we cancel any patients on *our specialty's* **elective lists**, to accommodate this patient?

   No

4. Do we have the *staffing* to safely open a **second emergency theatre**?

   No

5. Can we cancel patients on *another specialty's list*, to accommodate our patient?

   No

6. Is there a *suitable* **inter-hospital transfer** available? The patient must be stable, the receiving hospital must be within a reasonable distance and also have the capacity to perform the operation when the patient arrives.

At each stage, there should be early Consultant involvement and an MDT approach; it is not something that you, as a surgical trainee, will be managing on your own! Nevertheless, you should be able to demonstrate that you have an understanding of the options.

CHAPTER 14:

Knowledge-based interview stations

14.1: Apprenticeship

14.1.1: Capacity

Capacity is the ability to understand and use information to make a decision and, as a surgical trainee, you will be frequently faced with issues surrounding it.

The most essential aspects of capacity that you must have an awareness of are:
- how to **assess** capacity
- **when** to question a patient's capacity
- dealing with **incapacity**
- capacity in **children.**

Assessing capacity

To have capacity to make decisions about their care, a patient must demonstrate that they can:
1. understand the information
2. retain the information
3. utilise this information when making their decision
4. communicate the decision.

It is absolutely essential that, for all of the above criteria, you ensure that any necessary adjustments required to facilitate their fulfilment are made. These could include:

Criteria	Adjustments
Understand	• Use a level of vocabulary that is appropriate to the patient • Provide information in the correct language • Provide information in the format that they prefer (audio, written, pictures or other forms of media) • Frequently check the patient's understanding throughout the consultation
Retain	• Record the discussion in writing • Provide information booklets / leaflets / sheets
Utilise	• Give them time to consider the options • Allow the patient to have partners / friends / carers / advocates present, if they think it would help them make the decision
Communicate	• Allow their decision to be communicated to you in the format that they prefer

If they are unable to fulfil these criteria, despite all reasonable adjustments being made, then you should deem that the patient lacks capacity. Ensure that the consultation is carefully documented in the notes.

If you believe that there is significant uncertainty, and you do not feel that you can make the decision alone, a specialist opinion should be sought (from the psychiatrists, neurologists or other allied healthcare professionals).

Questioning capacity

The rules around questioning capacity are very simple:

You should not question a patient's capacity unless you have a reason to do so.

That is, the starting presumption is always that the patient *has* capacity and you should not question this "solely because of their age, disability, appearance, medical condition (including mental illness), beliefs, their apparent inability to communicate, or because they choose an option that you consider unwise" (GMC, 2020a).

The 'reason' to question a patient's capacity is therefore initially a subjective assessment that you make in the course of your dialogue with them. Should you find yourself questioning their capacity, formally assess it as described above.

Future capacity and advance statements

If a deterioration in the patient's capacity is foreseeable, it is reasonable to discuss future decisions whilst they still retain capacity. This ensures that future decisions are made in keeping with the patient's beliefs and can be made expeditiously, if needed.

Decisions could include:
- future treatment preferences
- treatments that they would refuse
- emergency interventions (including CPR) and ceiling of care
- who they would want to help make decisions on their behalf.

This is called an 'advance statement' and should be formalised legally, although it can of course be amended at any point.

Dealing with incapacity

Your response to incapacity will depend on a number of factors, described below.

The intervention can be safely delayed

- If the patient may regain their capacity and the decision can be safely delayed, then it should be.
- If there is no prospect of capacity being regained, then:
  - identify if the patient has previously expressed wishes about the decision in question, e.g. in an advance statement
  - identify if the patient has appointed someone to represent them (i.e. a 'lasting power of attorney').

When these are not available, the doctor is responsible for making the decision about what would be of 'overall benefit' to the patient. To assist in making this decision, you must:
- consider the patient's prior decisions and wishes
- liaise with the patient's close contacts – such as family members or healthcare workers (who know them well) – to understand the patient's previously expressed views
- select the treatment option that is least restrictive to their future decision-making, should they regain capacity.

The surgical interview

In an emergency
- If you have no reason to question the patient's capacity, then principles of consent remain the same.
- If they are incapacitated (e.g. due to unconsciousness or premorbid cognitive impairment):
  ○ if the intervention can be safely delayed, you should act as described in the paragraph above
  ○ if it cannot be safely delayed, you can provide emergency treatment to save their life or prevent significant morbidity.

Capacity in children

Assessing capacity in childhood is often actually quite simple but still causes much consternation amongst trainees. The broad principles are as follows, but you should have a **low threshold for seeking senior input.**
- From the age of 16, children can be presumed to have capacity and are therefore assessed as described for adults.
- Under 16, children may have capacity depending on maturity and their ability to understand what is involved – this is termed 'Gillick competence' (see box, below). Their understanding may vary significantly, especially if the intervention is going to have long-lasting consequences:
  A If a child *does not* have capacity:
    – A single parent's consent is sufficient
  B If a child *does* have capacity and *accepts* treatment:
    – Parents cannot override this
  C If a child *does* have capacity, but *refuses* treatment:
    – The law is complex as to whether the child's decision can be overridden. This is beyond the scope of the junior surgical trainee and urgent assistance should be sought from the paediatricians and legal experts.

Gillick competence

'Gillick competence' is the term used to describe if a child <16 years has the capacity to provide consent, without the need for parental knowledge or permission.

There is not a fixed set of questions; instead, the practitioner has to be satisfied that:
- the child understands the issue being discussed, including advantages, disadvantages and the long-term impact
- the child understands the benefits, risks and consequences of their decision
- they have a reasonable level of comprehension of any advice given
- they understand the alternatives
- they can clearly explain the rationale for their decision.

Broadly, the child must have sufficient maturity and judgement to enable them to fully understand what is proposed.

Practice questions

1. What four criteria must a patient meet to demonstrate capacity?
   a. Describe some adjustments you could employ to facilitate patients meeting these criteria.

2. For what reasons might you question a patient's capacity?

3. What would you recommend that a patient completes if they are likely to lose capacity in the near future?

4. In the incapacitated patient:
   a. Would you treat them in an emergency? What are the principles of this?
   b. How would you act if the treatment can be safely delayed?

5. Under what age is someone deemed a 'child'?
   a. What is 'Gillick competence' and how is it used?
   b. If a Gillick-competent child accepts a treatment, can their parents overrule this?

14.1.2: Consent

Stations that assess candidates' ability to obtain informed consent are common. The essential prerequisite is that:

> **To be able to give consent, you must have capacity**
> (Capacity is described fully in *Section 14.1.1*).

The surgical interview

What is consent?

Consent is the act of a patient granting permission to undergo a treatment or procedure. It reflects the fundamental right of patients to be involved in the decisions about their care, as outlined in international human rights law.

The process of gaining 'informed' consent is guided by seven principles, as described by the GMC (2020a):

1. All patients have a right to be involved in decisions about their care.
2. Decision making is an **ongoing process** based on meaningful dialogue.
3. All patients have the right to be listened to, and to be **given the information they need to make a decision** and the time and support they need to make it.
4. Doctors must try to find out what matters to the patient so they can **share relevant information about the benefits and harms of options and alternatives, including the option to take no action.**
5. Doctors must start from the presumption that all adult patients have capacity to make decisions about their treatment and care.
6. The choice of treatment or care for patients who lack capacity must be of overall benefit to them, and decisions should be made in consultation with those who are close to them or advocating for them.
7. Patients whose right to consent is affected by law should be supported to be involved in the decision-making process, and to exercise choice if possible.

Taking consent for a surgical intervention

These principles are used to shape how the consent process should be performed in clinical practice (and so in the interview).

Location
Consent should be obtained in the pre-assessment clinic and then confirmed on the morning of surgery.

Name of the procedure
State the name of the operation in both medical and lay terminology.

Description of the procedure
Describe the important steps of the procedure, to include:
- necessity for an anaesthetic and anaesthetic type
- incision location, orientation and size
- the main stages of the operation
- closure and dressings.

Alternatives, including to do nothing
Describe any viable alternative options, if there are any. Also always state that there is the option of doing nothing ('accepting the status quo') and explain the expected clinical outcome if this is pursued.

Benefits
State the intended benefit(s).

Risks
State the possible risks, their symptoms and treatment.

A helpful way of systematically describing the risks is by dividing them up into the main steps of the operation, as follows:

Stage of the operation	Associated risks

Incision	• Scarring:
	  o unsatisfactory cosmesis
	  o dehiscence
	  o surgical site infection

Dissection (the 'approach')	• Neurological injury • Vascular injury
Main operative intervention (specialty- and procedure-specific)	• These risks have to be learnt specifically – this includes risks associated with the specific operation, but also risks that are specific to that surgical specialty
Main operative intervention (general)	• Inadequacy or failure of the operation • Recurrence of the pathology
Postoperative period	• Pain • Stiffness • DVT / PE • Future surgery • MI / CVA / death

Adjunctive treatments or interventions
For example:
• blood transfusion, either from donor blood or autotransfusion
• surgical drains
• negative pressure dressings

- orthotics
- anaesthetic adjuncts such as lines, epidural catheters and PCA.

Postoperative care and anticipated recovery
Describe the 'routine' postoperative care that they should expect.

Summary
Concisely summarise the salient points of the procedure.

Questions
Provide ample time for questions.

Provision of written information
Where possible, provide written information that the patient can take away with them.

An example of informed consent

Candidates are often intimidated by this station, presumably because they do not regularly consent patients. Consequently, there is often a preoccupation with memorising the risks of various procedures, whilst completely ignoring the rest of the process; remember, marks are awarded for the *process* of consent, not just discussing the risks.

> **Clinical vignette:** a 24-year-old male due to undergo a right proximal femoral replacement for osteosarcoma of the femur.

Name of the procedure
You have attended the pre-assessment clinic today to discuss undergoing a right proximal femoral replacement – that is, replacing the top of the right thigh bone, as well as the right hip – to remove a cancer.

I'd like to begin by taking some time to describe what that involves, its benefits, risks and alternatives.

Description of the procedure
You will attend on the morning of surgery and again meet us, the surgical team, as well as the anaesthetic team. For this procedure, you will need to be asleep, so you will receive a general anaesthetic; the anaesthetists will describe this in more detail.

For the operation, we will make a curved incision on the outer aspect of the thigh and the back of the buttock. We then pass down through the layers of the body to reach your hip joint and the tumour. The tumour will be carefully removed, taking with it a thin layer of the normal tissues that surround it, so we increase the likelihood of removing it entirely. The tumour, along with the hip joint, is then removed. Following this, a combination of metal and plastic components are inserted to replace your hip joint.

Everything is then thoroughly cleaned, and the wound is closed with stitches, all of which are under the skin. You will have some dressings over the wound when you wake up.

Alternatives, including to do nothing
It is important that I let you know there are two alternatives to this operation; firstly, an amputation of the leg and, secondly, you can choose to decline surgery altogether. If this is the case, the cancer would be treated medically, meaning that there would be a lower chance of being cured; you would probably die as a consequence of this disease.

Benefits
The intention of the operation is to remove the cancer and replace your hip, so improving your pain and function.

Risks
However, as with all medical interventions, there are risks, and these include:

Incision
Surgical scarring which becomes unsightly or is slow to heal. Occasionally wounds will get infected, which would require antibiotic treatment and possibly further surgery.

Dissection
As we go through the layers of the body down to the hip, there is a slim chance of damaging the nerves or blood vessels. Nerves that are bruised give you pins and needles whilst they are recovering; rarely, a nerve is so badly injured it stops working altogether and is unlikely to recover. If a blood vessel is injured, this would be repaired whilst you are asleep.

Specialty- and procedure-specific risks
Regarding your hip replacement specifically, you may notice that your legs feel different lengths to begin with. Sometimes, joint replacements can pop out of the socket; this is called a dislocation and needs treatment in the emergency department. If it keeps happening, you would need further surgery to stabilise it. It's also important to remember that this hip replacement will not last for your lifetime and you will therefore need this operation again in the future.

General operative risks
All operations run the risk of not going as planned, so there is a chance that the cancer may come back with time.

Postoperative period
Once the operation is over, there are some further risks whilst you're recovering. You will be sore and stiff to begin with, so make sure you ask for plenty of pain relief. There is also a risk of blood clots in the legs or lungs; these need treating with blood thinners. Lastly, all surgery in general carries a slim risk of serious medical complications, such as heart attacks, strokes and death.

Adjunctive treatments or interventions
During the procedure you may need a blood transfusion – we can discuss this in more detail later.

When you wake up there may be a drain coming out of the wound; this is not painful and is removed after 24–48 hours. You will also have an epidural in your back, to give you good pain relief for the first few days after surgery.

Postoperative care and anticipated recovery
After the operation you will spend the first night on a high dependency ward, before moving back to the orthopaedic wards the following day. Once your pain is well controlled, the physiotherapists will work with you to help get you mobile again and, once you're safe on your feet, we will let you go home. This is usually a few nights or so.

We will need to see you back in the clinic in 2 weeks to make sure your wound is healing well.

Summary
To summarise, we're planning to do an operation to replace your hip and thigh bone in order to treat the cancer, with the intention of removing it completely, and improving your pain and function. There are a number of risks that we've discussed and I'll give you a leaflet about this to take home and read. We expect that you'll spend a few nights in hospital and we'll then see you back in a fortnight's time.

Questions
Is that clear? Do you have any questions that you would like to ask?

Practice questions

1. What is consent?

2. Describe some of the seven principles you should follow to aid the patient in making an 'informed' decision.

3. Broadly, what essential information should you provide when consenting a patient for a surgical intervention?
   a. What 'adjunctive treatments' might you mention?

4. What are some of the most common general risks of surgery, associated with:
   a. the incision?
   b. the dissection?
   c. the main operative intervention?
   d. the postoperative period?

14.1.3: Confidentiality

Confidentiality is at the heart of the doctor–patient relationship and the principles of confidentiality are frequently assessed at interview. A doctor is both **ethically** and **legally** bound to maintain confidentiality:

- **Ethically**, the trust a patient places in their doctor is partly dependent on the maintenance of confidentiality. If a patient cannot depend on confidentiality, they may under-present or under-report issues which they perceive to be embarrassing or in some other way deleterious to them if made public.
- **Legally**, you are bound to maintain confidentiality. The guidance differs over the four nations of the UK and a summary can be found here: www.gmc-uk. org/ethical-guidance/ethical-guidance-for-doctors/confidentiality/legal-annex.

What information is considered confidential?
Information or material which should be considered confidential includes:

- **identifying information**, such as name, identification number, location data or other factors specific to the patient (e.g. physical, physiological, genetic, economic, others)
- **health data**, such as case notes, test results, radiology results and correspondence.

Handling confidential information: the 'Caldicott principles'

The general way in which confidential information should be handled is dictated by the 'Caldicott principles'. These were outlined by Dame Fiona Caldicott following her review of patient information handling in 1997, and include the following tenets:

- **Use the minimum necessary information** and use anonymised information if feasible.
- **Protect information:** ensure personal information is handled with care at all times and protected against improper access, disclosure or loss.
- **Be aware of your responsibilities:** maintain an understanding of the principles of information governance.
- **Comply with the law:** all personal information must be handled lawfully.
- **Share relevant information** in line with these principles, unless the patient objects.
- **Seek explicit consent** to disclose patients' identifiable information for purposes other than their direct care or for local clinical audit (unless the disclosure is required by law or can be justified in the public interest).
- **Inform patients** about disclosures of personal information you make that they would not reasonably expect. Record your decisions to disclose / not disclose information.
- **Support patients to access their information.** Patients have legal rights to be informed about how their information is used. Respect their right to access their health records.

Disclosing confidential personal information

Confidentiality is not absolute, so you may breach it – if necessary – when the following circumstances apply:

- The patient consents to it, either *implicitly or explicitly*, for the sake of their **own** care or clinical audit.
- If you want to disclose their information for any reason **other than their own care** or clinical audit, *explicit* consent (either oral or written) is required.
- If the patient lacks capacity, you can disclose information if you believe it is in their overall benefit.
- The disclosure is required by law, or by a court order.
- Disclosure is justified in the public interest.
  - In general, maintaining confidentiality is in the overall public interest.
  - However, if a patient presents a risk of serious harm or communicable disease to the public, you may breach that patient's confidentiality in an attempt to reduce this risk.

> ### The 'Caldicott Guardian'
>
> **Where a novel or difficult decision needs to be taken about whether confidentiality should be breached, you should involve a 'Caldicott Guardian'.** This is a senior person within the organisation who is responsible for maintaining confidentiality and ensuring that patient information is used in accordance with the Caldicott principles.

> ### Practice questions
>
> 1. Why is maintaining confidentiality of benefit?
>
> 2. What information is considered confidential?
>
> 3. What 'principles' are described to help doctors handle patient information correctly?
>
> 4. Is disclosing patient information to another specialty – for example, if you're referring them – breaking confidentiality?
>
> 5. If the patient lacks capacity, in what circumstances can you break confidentiality?
>
> 6. In what situations can you break patient confidentiality?
>   a. If you're unsure, who could you contact?

14.1.4: Handover

What is handover?

The definition from the National Patient Safety Agency (NPSA) is "the transfer of professional responsibility and accountability for some or all aspects of care for a patient, or group of patients, to another person or professional group on a temporary or permanent basis".

> **Useful Resource:** *'Safe Handover: Safe Patients'* published by the BMA

Why is handover so common?

Due to the changes in the **working pattern of doctors** there has become a need for medical teams to transfer information – and thus clinical responsibility – between multiple teams **over the course of a single day**.

These changes to doctors' contracts resulted in the following:

- A move towards **shift work**, as the number of hours a doctor can work consecutively has been limited.

The surgical interview

- **Multiple** teams looking after the **same** group of patients over a day. For example, it will usually be the Consultant's Firm looking after the patient between 8am and 5pm, the specialty doctor on-call between 5pm and 8pm and the 'Hospital at Night' team overnight. It is worth noting that the overnight teams rarely include specialty doctors.
- The teams looking after patients out of hours have **rarely ever had contact with the patients that they are caring for**.

Consequently, there are typically three (or sometimes more) handovers per patient, per day.

Why is handover important?
The central adage is "continuity of information underlies continuity of care" (BMA, 2004). Any discontinuity in care **endangers patient safety**.

How can safe handover be achieved?

System changes	The handover process
• Ensure there is adequate **time in the rota** for handover • Have a specific **time and location** for handover • Ensure that there are easy-access **computer systems** • Ensure that **up-to-date clinical information** for all patients being handed over is available and readily accessible	• **Supervised** by a senior clinician • **Succinct and pertinent information** is presented only • **Clinically unstable patients are highlighted** to the senior doctors • Outstanding tasks are highlighted to junior doctors and **their importance understood** • **Anticipated** problems are highlighted

Actions after handover
Handover is only of value if, after handover has been taken, the receiving team **form a robust, collective plan to act on the information provided**. This should involve the prioritisation of tasks and delegation of responsibilities and jobs.

Practice questions
1. What is 'handover' and why is it important?
2. Why is handover becoming increasingly common?
3. In what ways can the effectiveness of handover be increased?
4. What should happen after handover?

14.1.5: Triage

What is triage?

The word 'triage' is from the French for *'to sort'* or *'to grade'*. It was in the late 18th century that the triage process was pioneered in the context of warfare and mass casualties.

In medicine, it is the process of using readily available, quantitative parameters (such as basic observations) to *sort* the patient into a category of urgency; this allows them to be **prioritised by clinical need**.

When is triage required?

Triage is required when clinical need exceeds the available capacity. Consequently, the need for triage is inherent to working within healthcare. Whilst most obvious within the ED, where there is a formal triage process, doctors are continuously triaging clinical information to help them prioritise tasks.

Within surgery, **the triage of surgical patients has been formalised using the following**:

> National Confidential Enquiry into Patient Outcome and Death (NCEPOD): classification of intervention

NCEPOD: classification of intervention

Surgical cases are classified into one of the following four groups:

1. *Immediate* – an immediately life-, limb- or organ-saving intervention. Surgery happens within **minutes** of the decision to operate.
   - Examples include ruptured abdominal aortic aneurysms (rAAAs), major trauma to the thorax or abdomen, major neurovascular deficit, compartment syndrome.

2. *Urgent* – a potentially life- or limb-threatening condition, or for the control of distressing symptoms. Surgery happens within **hours** of the decision.
   - Examples include fractures, bowel perforations, critical ischaemia.

3. *Expedited* – The condition is *not* imminently life- or limb-threatening but requires early treatment. Surgery happens within **days**.
   - Examples include tendon and nerve injuries, and many other surgical interventions in a stable, non-septic patient.

4. *Elective* – Not life- or limb-threatening. Surgery is scheduled to **ensure timing is optimal** for the patient, staff and hospital.
   * All other conditions.

By categorising your patient into one of these groups, it will ensure that:
* patients are allocated to the **correct** surgical lists (i.e. out-of-hours vs. daytime lists)
* patients are operated on **within a window that is appropriate** for their condition
* the **running order** of 'emergency' operating lists is appropriate for the clinical urgency of the case.

Up to 25% of total operating is constituted by non-elective cases (particularly in T&O, Neurosurgery, General surgery, Vascular, Plastics and Transplant), so the ability to properly triage surgical cases is essential.

Hot topic: Out-of-hours operating

In 2003, the NCEPOD published their report *'Who Operates When? II'*. It recommended that less *non-emergency* operative work was performed out of hours and that all operations for non-life- and non-limb-threatening conditions are completed before midnight.

The rationale for this is as follows:
* The overnight theatre **staff may be less experienced** in the use of specialty-specific equipment.
* There is **less availability of other staff** overnight, such as radiographers, laboratory staff and porters.
* The surgical intervention is **more likely to be undertaken by trainee surgeons**, who may underestimate the severity of the patient's condition or take on work beyond their competence.
* These cases are more likely to be **time-critical**.
* Doctors working on-call may have been working for many hours and **so may be excessively tired.**

The current standards in surgery are in keeping with these recommendations. Emergency operating lists are now *scheduled daily*, there is often a *'twilight'* operating list which accommodates urgent cases (but is finished before midnight) and there is *more readily available consultant support* overnight.

Practice questions

1. What is triage and why is it required in healthcare?

2. In surgery, what classification is used to triage the urgency of a case?
   a. What are the 4 classifications?
   b. Describe each and give an example of a clinical condition that falls into that category.
   c. Why not just perform all operations at the earliest possible time?

3. Are you aware of any guidelines about operating after midnight?
   a. What is the rationale for recommending that all non-life- and non-limb-threatening procedures are completed before this time?

Resource: www.ncepod.org.uk/2003report/Downloads/03full.pdf

14.1.6: Patient safety

Patient safety is a central principle for healthcare delivery; we are obligated to **first, do no harm**.

Broadly, patient safety can be achieved in three ways:
1. **Prior** to the delivery of healthcare
2. **During** the delivery of healthcare
3. Through processes that allow us to **learn from** adverse events, to protect patient safety in the future.

Prior to healthcare delivery
Education and training are the central component of ensuring patient safety prior to the delivery of healthcare. Examples include:
- **Medical school and postgraduate training** – rigorous selection methods and assessment to ensure everyone meets a minimum standard.
- **Professional development** – receiving up-to-date evidence-based teaching and training; attending conferences and courses; general engagement in the medical community.
- **Governance** – the development of national and local policies, protocols and guidelines.
- **Research** – clinical trials and studies to ensure therapeutic options offered to patients are safe.

During healthcare delivery
Safety processes are built into the delivery of healthcare:

- **Pre-procedure checks** – three forms of identification (name, date of birth, hospital number); the 'surgical pause' / WHO Surgical Checklist; gaining informed consent.

WHO Surgical Safety Checklist

Take some time to read through the WHO surgical safety checklist and understand why the questions asked are included.

An example checklist can be found here: www.england.nhs.uk/2019/01/surgical-safety-checklist/

- **Prescribing** – protocols and guidelines; standardised drug names (i.e. no trade names); dosage calculators; restricted medications.
- **Clinical procedures** – regular baseline observations using standardised charts; 'early warning scores' with protocolised escalation requirements depending on the patient score; standardised escalation policies; standardised emergency procedures.
- **Culture** – we have a duty to raise concerns when they arise (as per the GMC).

Resource – *'Ethical guidance for doctors'* by the General Medical Council

The GMC mandates that we must "promote and encourage a culture that allows staff to raise concerns openly and safely".

More can be read here: www.gmc-uk.org/ethical-guidance/ethical-guidance-for-doctors/raising-and-acting-on-concerns/about-this-guidance

Learning from safety issues

It is essential that we learn from issues that arise, so as to diminish the risk of them occurring again in the future. There are many methods of doing this, some of which are mandatory in surgical training:

- **Incident reporting** – the National Patient Safety Agency (NPSA) *mandates* that healthcare professionals must "report any unintended or unexpected incidents which could have, or did, lead to harm". This allows all adverse events to be investigated and understood (see *Section 14.1.7*, Adverse event management).
- **Audit** – audit is used to understand if the healthcare that is being provided is in line with the accepted national standards. Performing an audit is a core requirement of surgical training.
- **Quality improvement (QI)** – this is the process of attempting to improving the safety and effectiveness of healthcare provision, by applying wide-ranging methodology (such as 'plan-do-study-act (PDSA), cycles or 'Six Sigma').

> Resource for understanding QI principles: www.health.org.uk/publications/
> quality-improvement-made-simple

- **Root cause analysis (RCA)** – this is a systematic method for understanding
  the fundamental underlying cause(s) of an adverse event, commonly
  utilised in healthcare and other industries. When used correctly, it has been
  demonstrated to reduce the incidence of surgical errors.

Practice questions

1. Prior to the delivery of healthcare, what actions help to maintain patient safety?

2. Prior to starting an operation, what actions are undertaken to maintain
   patient safety?
   a. What is included on the 'surgical pause'?
   b. What is the intention of the surgical 'sign out'?

3. In what ways can we learn from patient safety issues?

14.1.7: Adverse event management

An adverse event (AE) is any event that "could have caused, or did result in, harm
to people or groups of people", where 'harm' is "an outcome with a negative effect"
(Healthcare Improvement Scotland, 2019). Therefore, there is an expectation, cited in
Good Medical Practice, that "all doctors will, whatever their role, take appropriate action
to raise and act on concerns about patient care, dignity and safety". (GMC, 2020c).

There are six stages of adverse event management (Healthcare Improvement
Scotland, 2019):

Stage	Description
1: Risk assessment and prevention	Organisations should foster a culture of openness and fairness, where reporting and learning from incidents is the norm. This is termed a 'positive safety culture'.
2: Identification and immediate actions	The first action following an AE is to ensure the patient is attended to, with the aim to minimise the impact of the event. The environment in which the AE occurred should be made safe, so normal activities can resume promptly. The team has a duty of candour to be open and honest with the patient about what has happened.

Stage	Description
3: Initial reporting and notification	All hospitals have electronic reporting systems for AEs. A comprehensive description of the event should be completed on the system, as close as possible to when it occurred.
4: Assessment and categorisation	There are three categories of AE: • **Category 1**: resulted in *permanent* harm • **Category 2**: resulted in *temporary* harm • **Category 3**: had the *potential* to cause harm, but no harm occurred (termed a 'near miss').
5: Review and analysis	A comprehensive review of the incident is performed in order to identify learning points, which may be applicable locally, regionally or nationally. It aims to establish *what* happened, *how* it happened and *why* it happened.
6: Improvement planning and monitoring	The learning points from an AE review should be formulated into an improvement plan, and then implemented in order to avoid the same event happening again. These should be reviewed and appraised regularly.

Interview questions

All AEs questioned at interview will be individual with respect to the level of harm and the people involved; however, you can use the broad principles described above to structure a generic answer. These can be assimilated into the following:

Understand the **ISSUE**

and

Manage the **RISK**

Understand the ISSUE
Information
- Seek information on:
  - the patient's clinical condition, as this is your first concern
  - the environment in which the AE occurred, as you need to ensure that it is safe in order to avoid immediate further harm
  - the event, as you will need to report it in due course.

Safety
- If harm has occurred, the patient's current clinical care is your primary concern.
- If there is risk of ongoing harm, either to the current patient or another patient, this will also need addressing.

Significance
- This will be determined by an AE review.

UrgEncy
- Category 1 and 2 AEs require immediate action, whereas Category 3 AEs should be dealt with at your earliest convenience.

Manage the RISK

Recommendation and Referral
- The AE will need electronically reporting and a review panel will deal with the issues.
- The question is really about *who* should log the incident report.

Intervention
- Provide immediate medical care to the patient, to reduce the impact of the AE.
- Liaise with the rest of the team to ensure the environment in which it occurred is made safe, to prevent further harm.
- The incident should be electronically reported as close to the time it happened as is feasible and should include as much detail as possible.
- Our duty of candour mandates that we must be open and honest with the patient about the event.

Substitution
- If you are needed to attend to the incident, and are therefore unable to undertake your scheduled activity, arrange suitable cover.

Knowledge
- It is essential that lessons are learnt from the AE.
  - Incident reporting facilitates this by permitting a panel to review the AE and to understand what happened, and how and why it happened.
  - It allows the formulation of learning points, which should be implemented at a local, regional or national level (depending on the incident).
  - These learning points require ongoing review and appraisal.
- Write a reflective portfolio entry about the event and how you responded to it, to improve your future performance.

The surgical interview

> ### Never events
>
> A 'never event' is a "serious, largely preventable patient safety incident that **should not occur** if healthcare providers have implemented **existing** national guidance or safety recommendations" (NHS Improvement, 2018).
>
> In surgery, there are three types of never event:
> * wrong site surgery
> * wrong implant / prosthesis
> * retained foreign objects post procedure

> ### Practice questions
>
> 1. What is an 'adverse event' in healthcare?
>
> 2. What should your immediate action be?
>
> 3. When should the incident report be completed?
>
> 4. How are adverse events categorised?
>   a. If no harm occurred, but the event had the potential to do so, what is this termed?
>   b. What is a 'never event'? Name the three that are specific to surgery.

14.1.8: Order of escalation

Choosing **who** to speak with about a specific problem is an important, yet often undervalued, skill. You can divide the principles of escalation into 'non-clinical' and 'clinical'.

Non-clinical order of escalation

When you are required to escalate a non-clinical issue (e.g. ethical dilemmas or probity issues), you must ensure that you escalate only to the *lowest possible grade of doctor that is required to fully resolve the issue*. Escalating disproportionately can be very damaging in many ways.

> Note: in almost all instances, it is preferable to encourage the colleague to escalate an issue themselves in the first instance. If they are not willing to do this, you should escalate the issue; however, you do not wish to be seen as 'going behind their back', so **you must inform them** that you are going to be escalating the issue, prior to doing so.

A sensible order of escalation is as follows:

- A senior colleague:
  - In general, it is best to first discuss these sorts of issues with a senior colleague who is not in the same tier as you. This avoids gossip amongst your near-peers, which can be harmful.
  - Furthermore, you may wish to avoid discussing an issue with members of that person's team in the first instance, as this may lead to your colleague losing face amongst them.
- A Consultant (yours or theirs):
  - Think carefully if you need to involve the Consultant as, more often than not, issues can be resolved without the input of very senior staff.
  - You may wish to discuss the issue with your Consultant, in confidence, prior to discussing the issue with the person's Consultant. They can often offer excellent insight and advice to help you resolve the issues appropriately; furthermore, they may be happy to take over from you in dealing with the issue.
- A clinical supervisor (yours or theirs)
- An educational supervisor (yours or theirs)
- The Training Programme Director (TPD): this is the last point of call as, in informing their TPD, you may affect their future training progression. It would be essential that you have sought counsel from a number of people before you inform the TPD of an issue.

> **Tip: Raising concerns about a Consultant**
>
> When raising concerns about a Consultant, you should consider seeking counsel from someone **outside your unit**, in the first instance. This can be very helpful in providing an objective assessment of the situation, avoiding gossip and helping to save face.

Clinical order of escalation

Where the clinical question is not an emergency, the order of escalation should be:

- A near-peer:
  - If one of your colleagues is nearby, asking them if they know the answer should be your first port of call.
- The seniors on your team:
  - Generally, contact them in ascending grade order.
- The on-call Registrar:
  - If your team is unavailable and the question cannot wait, the on-call registrar may be able to help.

The surgical interview

- The team's Consultant:
  - You can contact Consultants on their personal phones via the hospital switchboard. If the answer cannot wait for the other members of your team to become available, call the Consultant.
- The on-call Consultant:
  - This is the last point of call for any question which cannot wait.

Tip: Referral to specialty

When referring to specialty for a pre-existing condition, it is generally accepted that you contact the named Consultant's team from that specialty first, rather than referring to the on-call team.

For example, if you want advice on the peri-operative management for a patient with cystic fibrosis, contact the *named* Consultant from respiratory medicine who ordinarily sees the patient in clinic (rather than calling the on-call respiratory Registrar).

14.1.9: Challenging consultations

As a surgical trainee you will inevitably encounter challenging consultations, often concerning difficult or emotive topics. Consequently, **a candidate's ability to manage a challenging consultation is a frequent component of the surgical interview**. Such stations are generally an observed consultation with a simulated patient but may also form the basis of a hypothetical discussion with the interviewer.

N.B. It is common for the first half of a clinical station to be 'knowledge' based (e.g. 'can you consent this patient for a DHS?'), followed by a second half that is a challenging consultation (often as a result of a surgical complication).

These situations are complex and managing them effectively requires experience and sensitivity, as well as the application of theoretical knowledge.

Principles for managing challenging consultations

Although these scenarios are usually unique, having been designed specifically for the interview, there are some general techniques which are useful to know and to practise:

1. Gain personal emotional control

This means controlling your own emotions before engaging with another. No scenario (in interview or reality) occurs in a vacuum; internal and external factors play an important role, and entering the situation in a calm, positive and composed manner sets the tone for the interaction.

> **Interview tips**
>
> - Be calm before entering the consultation; counteract your own 'fight or flight' response.
> - Be proactive – approach the situation on your terms.
> - Know your triggers, recognise them and control your reaction.

2. Make a good first impression

- As with all interactions, first impressions count. Positively shaping someone's initial perception of you can set the tone that you hope to continue throughout the engagement. People are human; it's rather more difficult to be aggressive to someone who is projecting a calm, pleasant demeanour.

> **Interview tips**
>
> - Smile and present a mild manner.
> - Maintain good eye contact and open body language.
> - Be pleasant; strike an amiable but sincere tone.

3. Help the patient gain emotional control

- The patient may be 'primed' with anger, fear or anxiety: if you can defuse this initial emotion at the outset, then you can set the tone for the conversation.

> **Interview tips**
>
> - Adopt a calm approach.
> - Reassure them that their issue will be taken seriously and addressed, e.g. *"I'm here to help you".*
> - Give them a chance to get things 'off their chest', e.g. *"I'm going to listen to what you want to say, and then we can talk through this together".*

4. Empathetic listening

- Many difficult consultations arise when a patient feels a lack of autonomy, either because of a medical situation or because they feel that their concerns aren't being considered. Being listened to is an extremely reassuring feeling in times of fear or anxiety. Demonstrate that you are concerned about their feelings and wish to share their perspective, however unreasonable you think it may be.

The surgical interview

Interview tips

- Demonstrate 'active listening' with nodding, eye contact and appropriate acknowledgements.
- Allow the patient time to speak; try not to make them feel rushed.
- If the patient is irate, use judicious pauses to allow them to 'burn out' and lose momentum.
- Acknowledge emotion. A sincere "I can see that you are upset" can go a long way.

Practice stations

1. Following an attempted closed reduction of a shoulder dislocation, the post-procedure X/R demonstrates a fracture of the surgical neck of the humerus.

2. At their 3-month follow-up clinic, a patient has florid keloid scarring on their chest following a median sternotomy.

3. You are called to see a patient's free flap at 2am; it is clear that it is threatened and requires emergency exploration in theatre.

4. A patient is on prophylactic dalteparin postoperatively. They attend A&E with a large haemarthrosis and are unable to weight-bear.

5. A 24-year-old man attends the urology clinic with a urethral stricture, following a traumatic attempted catheterisation in A&E 6 months earlier.

6. A patient is in orthopaedic outpatients demanding a hip replacement for their 'hip' pain; it is quite clear that their pain is originating from their lower back.

7. The son of one of your postoperative patients attends the ward asking for an update; however, the patient has explicitly told you not to share his clinical information with the son, but asks that you don't reveal that to him. The son is getting increasingly angry.

14.2: Leadership

14.2.1: Responsibilities in the workplace

As with all doctors, a surgeon's primary responsibility is the care and safety of patients. Many of the surgical workplace responsibilities are covered in more detail elsewhere in this book, but it's worth looking in detail at specific guidance produced by the GMC (2020b) in the section *Duties of a doctor in the workplace*. The principles can be summarised as follows:

Principle	Description
Patient-centred approach	Commitment to delivering a 'patient-centred' approach to healthcare. This principle is at the heart of organisational mission statements, stated responsibilities and training curriculums. It places consideration of the patient foremost in all decisions and processes.
Engagement with colleagues	Engage with colleagues and work to deliver care as active participants of MDTs. Develop and maintain effective team-working and leadership skills.
Improvement and safety	Participate in discussions around improvement and raise concerns about safety.
Fairness and inclusivity	Work in a manner which promotes fairness and inclusivity, and prohibits unfair discrimination against staff, patients or the public.
Medical education	Continued engagement in teaching and training is a central tenet in medicine, which is not just limited to formal medical education commitments – this is reflected in the Hippocratic Oath and modern derivatives.
Efficiency	Resources should be used in an efficient and justifiable manner. Surgeons have a duty to their patients and to the population as a collective – this should be considered when allocating and expending resources (e.g. time, equipment, staff).

14.2.2: Ethical principles

Developing an understanding of ethics and professionalism begins before medical school and runs throughout a surgeon's career. To most people, much of this will appear to be 'common sense' and may be given less attention than other topics. Remember – a sound ethical framework and the maintenance of rigorous professionalism is essential for doctors at every stage, and because of this you will encounter formal assessment of your own standards in any interview and at every stage in your career.

The four *prima facie* principles of biomedical ethics are:

1. **Non-maleficence** – first, do no harm *(primum non nocere)*
   An intervention must do no harm to the patient or to society. This fundamental principle is ancient and essential, but is more nuanced than absolute. All surgery causes some degree of harm; what is important is that this **harm must not be unacceptable, inappropriate or disproportionate** to the intentions of the treatment.

2. **Beneficence** – act in the best interest of the patient
   A treatment or healthcare intervention must be made with the intent of doing good by the patient or society. This will not be the same for all patients (therefore consideration of the individual is important), nor will it be the same for all interventions.

3. **Autonomy** – the patient has the right to choose
   The patient should be allowed to make decisions regarding their health wherever possible, and in a decision-making process which puts them at the centre. Autonomy is contingent upon complex issues of capacity, competence and consent.

4. **Justice** – Patients must be treated fairly (allocation of treatments / resources)
   Healthcare must be distributed in a manner which is fair and just. This pertains to the allocation of treatments and resources, as well as the design and delivery of systems such as an individual surgeon's practice, through to national healthcare systems.

These four principles are fundamental pillars in medical ethics; however, they are not absolute and must be taken within the broader context of ethical considerations. A dilemma arises when two or more of these principles clash, and solving these requires understanding and experience. Broadly speaking, the principle of autonomy usually prevails when these ethical challenges arise.

14.3: Scholarship

14.3.1: Statistical definitions

Statistical definitions are **commonly examined in surgical interviews** and they are easy marks to pick up. As a surgical trainee there is a requirement over your training to publish in the literature, so it is important that you are confident in the application of basic statistical definitions.

P-value ('calculated probability')

The P-value is the probability of finding an observed result, when the null hypothesis is true. This can be described as *'the likelihood that the result you have observed is **due to chance**'*.

The smaller the P-value, the stronger the evidence is in favour of your observed result. The significance level at which you reject the null hypothesis is conventionally set at 5% (P <0.05).

Example:
- **Result**: a study gives a relative risk of 1.6 (null hypothesis value = 1.0) and the statistical test provides a P-value of 0.025.
- **Meaning**: there is a 2.5% likelihood that the result of 1.6 is due to chance. This falls below the conventionally set level of 5% and so we therefore reject the null hypothesis; we can assume that result of 1.6 is a true result and did not occur due to chance.

Type 1 (α) and type 2 (β) statistical errors

Type 1 and type 2 statistical errors recognise that error is an integral part of statistical testing.

1. **Type 1 (α) error**:
   - Finding a **'false positive'**.
   - You reject the null hypothesis when it is actually true.
   - **It is influenced by the P-value**; the smaller the P-value, the smaller the chance of finding a type 1 error. For example, if you set your significance level at 5% (P = 0.05), then you have a 5% chance of falsely rejecting the null hypothesis, whereas if you set P = 0.01 there is only a 1% chance.
   - It is influenced by the **number of tests** that you perform on your data. For example, if you performed 20 tests then, by chance, you would expect 1 result (5%) to be due to chance – this is a 'false positive' = a type 1 error.

2. **Type 2 (β) error**:
   - Finding a **'false negative'**.
   - You accept the null hypothesis when it is actually false.
   - This value (termed 'β') is usually set at 0.2: *there is a 20% chance that you will miss an association when in fact there is a true difference present*.
   - It is influenced by the **sample size** – the larger the sample size, the lower the chance of finding a 'false negative'.

The 'power' of a test

Type 2 (β) error is used to define the 'power' of a test, where **power = 1 – β**.

The 'power' is usually therefore 0.8 (= 80%).

'Power' is the chance of finding a result of a specific *magnitude*. Let's say there is a 25% reduction in the incidence of an outcome after a new treatment. If the power is 0.8, then there is an 80% chance of finding a difference *of that magnitude* (i.e. of 25%).

Confidence interval (CI)

This is the range of values within which there is a 95% chance that the **'true'** result lies. If this range does not include the null hypothesis value, then the null hypothesis is rejected.

Example:
- **Result**: a study gives a relative risk of an event happening of 1.4 (CI 1.25–1.65, P = 0.03).
- **Meaning**: there is a 95% chance that the 'true' value is somewhere between 1.25 and 1.65 (as the CI is 1.25–1.65). The probability of this being due to chance is 3% (as the P-value is 0.03). The null hypothesis value is 1.0 and we can therefore reject it.

Prevalence, incidence and incidence rate

These terms should not be confused.

Prevalence is **existing cases**:

$$Prevalence = \left(\frac{Number\, of\, cases}{Total\, population} \right) \times 100$$

Incidence is **new cases**:

$$Incidence = \left(\frac{New\, cases}{Total\, population} \right) \times 100$$

The incidence *rate* is the frequency of **new cases** over a specified time period. The result is usually given as 'X number of cases per 1000 person-years':

$$Incidence = \left(\frac{New\, cases\, over\, 'n'\, years}{Total\, population\, at\, risk\, over\, 'n'\, years} \right) \times 1000$$

Relative risk (RR)

This is how much more likely a group is to have an outcome if exposed to something, when compared to the unexposed group. An RR >1 indicates that those exposed are more likely to develop the outcome compared to those that were unexposed. It is based on the **incidence**.

	Event occurred	Event absent
Exposed	a	b
Unexposed	c	d

So, the chance of an event *occurring* if:

- you're exposed $= \dfrac{a}{(a+b)}$
- you're unexposed $= \dfrac{c}{(c+d)}$

So the RR is $= \dfrac{Chance\ of\ developing\ the\ outcome\ if\ exposed}{Chance\ of\ developing\ the\ outcome\ unexposed} = \dfrac{\frac{a}{(a+b)}}{\frac{c}{(c+d)}} = \dfrac{a(c+d)}{c(a+b)}$

Odds ratio (OR)

This is a measure of the odds of an outcome in an exposed vs. unexposed group. If the OR >1 then the chance of the outcome occurring is higher following the exposure.

The 'odds' of something occurring within a group (i.e. exposed vs. unexposed) is the:

$$\frac{Number\ of\ events}{Number\ of\ non\text{-}events}$$

Using the table above, OR can be described as follows:

$$\frac{\begin{array}{c}Odds\ of\ the\ event\\in\ exposed\ group\end{array}}{\begin{array}{c}Odds\ of\ the\ event\ in\\unexposed\ group\end{array}} = \frac{\left(\dfrac{Number\ of\ events\ in\ exposed\ group}{Number\ of\ non\text{-}events\ in\ exposed\ group}\right)}{\left(\dfrac{Number\ of\ events\ in\ unexposed\ group}{Number\ of\ non\text{-}events\ in\ unexposed\ group}\right)} = \frac{\left(\dfrac{a}{b}\right)}{\left(\dfrac{c}{d}\right)} = \frac{ad}{bc}$$

The surgical interview

Relative risk (RR) vs. odds ratio (OR)

As you can see, both the RR and OR are calculated from the same table of results.

RR is the likelihood of an outcome happening in relation to **all possible outcomes**. You know the exposure and then look to see if the outcome develops or not. Subsequently, it is based on the incidence and is therefore a **ratio of probabilities**. It can therefore be utilised in cohort studies.

OR compares events with non-events. You know the outcome, then look retrospectively to see if the person was exposed or unexposed. The OR is therefore a **ratio of ratios**. It is useful in case-control studies.

Where the number of participants is large and the outcome is rare, RR and OR are similar and so can be used interchangeably. However, if the outcome is common, OR exaggerates the effect of the exposure and so should be avoided.

Characteristics of diagnostic tests

The below terms are used frequently in clinical medicine so should be fully understood. All of the terms can be calculated using the following table:

		'True' diagnosis	
		Diagnosis present	Diagnosis absent
Test result	Positive	a	b
	Negative	c	d

1. **Sensitivity** – if the disease is present, the likelihood that the test is positive

$$= \frac{a}{(a+c)}$$

2. **Specificity** – if the disease is absent, the likelihood that the test is negative

$$= \frac{b}{(b+d)}$$

3. **Positive predictive value (PPV)** – if the test is positive, the chance that the diagnosis is also present

$$= \frac{a}{(a+b)}$$

4. **Negative predictive value (NPV)** – if the test is negative, the chance that the diagnosis is also absent

$$= \frac{d}{(c+d)}$$

In routine clinical practice:
- diagnostic tests need a high sensitivity and specificity
- screening tests require a high PPV and NPV.

Practice questions

1. What is the P-value? Describe it in lay terms.
   a. What value is it typically set at? What does this mean?

2. What is a type 1 statistical error?
   a. What factors influence it?

3. What is a type 2 statistical error?
   a. What value is it typically set at?
   b. What factors influence it?
   c. How is it related to the 'power' of a test?

4. Define the confidence interval.

5. How do prevalence and incidence differ?

6. What is the difference between the relative risk and the odds ratio?

7. What are the four characteristics of a diagnostic test?
   a. Draw a table to demonstrate how they're each calculated.
   b. How do they influence (i) screening tests and (ii) diagnostic tests?

14.3.2: Study designs

An appreciation of the types of study design, their uses, qualities and limitations is commonly tested in surgical interviews.

Levels of evidence

The term 'level' of evidence is routinely used in medicine. It is a system utilised to **hierarchically classify the *quality* of evidence**, with level 1 being the highest quality and level 4 being the poorest quality.

The surgical interview

The levels of evidence are set out in the below table, as described by the Oxford Centre for Evidence-Based Medicine (2009):

Level	Therapy / Prevention, Aetiology / Harm
1a	Systematic Review (with homogeneity) of Randomised Controlled Trials
1b	Individual Randomised Controlled Trial (with narrow Confidence Interval)
1c	All or none
2a	Systematic Review (with homogeneity) of cohort studies
2b	Individual cohort study (including low quality Randomised Controlled Trial; e.g. <80% follow-up)
2c	"Outcomes" Research; Ecological studies
3a	Systematic Review (with homogeneity) of case-control studies
3b	Individual Case-Control Study
4	Case-series (and poor quality cohort and case-control studies)

In turn, the 'level' of evidence available for a particular intervention can be **used to 'grade' the strength of the recommendation to support that intervention**. For example, if a recommendation for a treatment is given a grade A (strong recommendation), there will have been level 1 evidence (or consistent, multiple findings from level 2/3/4) supporting it.

Randomised controlled trials

Randomised controlled trials (RCTs) are *experimental* studies and are considered the gold standard for evaluating clinical interventions, particularly where the benefit may be small or offset by inadvertent harm. They will generally compare the current best-practice intervention with a new intervention, although there are many different study designs.

Strengths	Limitations
Randomisation essentially removes confounding and selection bias	They are expensive and logistically difficult to undertake
Blinding reduces performance and assessment bias	There may be difficulty in recruiting patients
Prospective collection of data removes recall bias	The participants may not mirror the 'real-life' group of patients, so applicability of results could be affected

The common biases in RCTs are:

- Selection bias – this is where randomisation is lost because the person recruiting is not fully blinded and therefore selectively recruits people that they think are 'suitable' for inclusion.
- Performance bias – this is where there is a systematic difference in the care that groups receive; again, due to inadequate blinding.
- Detection bias – this bias is where there is a systematic difference in a way that the outcomes for the groups are assessed.
- Attrition bias – this is where there has been a systematic difference in the number of patients that have withdrawn from the study groups.

Phases of randomised controlled trials

When assessing the effectiveness of a new intervention, trials go through different 'phases':

- **Phase 1:** a small number of patients are given the drug at a very limited dose
  - Purpose: to assess safety, pharmacokinetics and pharmacodynamics
- **Phase 2:** a larger number of patients are recruited and the drug is given at a higher, therapeutic dose
  - Purpose: to demonstrate efficacy and dosing
- **Phase 3:** large groups of patients are recruited and randomised to intervention or no intervention
  - Purpose: the definitive assessment of the clinical effectiveness of the intervention
- **Phase 4:** this is the 'post-marketing' phase, where the effects of the intervention are monitored over time
  - Purpose: to detect rare or long-term sequelae

The surgical interview

> **Issues with RCTs in surgery** (adapted from Wartolowska *et al.*, 2016)
>
> There are many issues with performing RCTs in surgery, meaning that only around a quarter of surgical interventions are based on evidence from RCTs. These include:
> - high cost and challenges with funding
> - challenges with blinding; often, neither the patient nor surgeon can be blinded
> - different levels of experience in the operating surgeons
> - high degrees of variability in the patients
> - challenges with delivering a placebo; for example, is it ethical to perform 'sham' surgery – where an operation is performed, but the 'therapeutic' part is withheld in the placebo group?
> - uncertainty over the best way to assess surgical outcomes.

Cohort studies

Cohort studies are observational studies that come in two forms:
- Prospective: these begin by identifying a group of people who *do not* have the outcome of interest – people are then **classified by an exposure** (exposed vs. unexposed) and followed up over time, **to see if they develop the outcome of interest**.
- Retrospective: these begin by identifying people with a particular **exposure** and then look retrospectively at their medical records to identify if they, *at any point in the past*, had developed the outcome of interest. In this group, **both** the exposure *and* the outcome of interest **have already occurred**.

Strengths	Limitations
Good for investigating rare exposures	Prospective studies are expensive and require long periods of follow-up
Can examine multiple outcomes for a single exposure	Attrition bias possible in prospective studies
Causality can be assessed, and the sequence of events can be determined	Retrospective studies prone to recall bias

(Table adapted from Song and Chung, 2010).

Common biases:
- Selection bias – this occurs where the exposed and unexposed patients are selected from systematically different groups. To minimise this, both should come from the same source.

- Attrition bias – this is where patients are lost over time due to the length of the follow-up period.

Case-control studies

Case-control studies, like cohort studies, are also observational studies. Whereas cohort studies begin by identifying patients with a specific exposure, case-control studies identify patients with a specific **outcome of interest** (the 'cases'). A 'control' group (i.e. people *without* the outcome) are then identified; it is essential that they are drawn from the same source group. Investigators then look retrospectively to identify who, within both the 'cases' and 'controls', were exposed or unexposed to something of interest.

Strengths	Limitations
Good for investigating rare outcomes	Difficult to select a representative 'control' group
Cheap and relatively quick	Cannot calculate rates of disease
	Prone to recall bias and interviewer bias

(Table adapted from Song and Chung, 2010).

Common biases:

- Recall bias: all data is collected retrospectively, often by interview/questionnaire. It is possible that those with the outcome of interest are more likely to say that they did have the exposure, also.
- Interviewer bias: as the interviewer knows the outcome, it is possible that they unintentionally ask leading questions which encourage patients with the outcome of interest to state that they were exposed. Collectively, recall and interviewer bias can cause the study to **overestimate** the importance of the exposure.

> **Useful resource:** *Observational studies: cohort and case-control studies* by Song and Chung, 2010. See *References*.

Case series

These are typically small, descriptive studies that identify patients with a specific exposure and look at their outcomes over time. They sound similar to a cohort study; however, a case series has **no unexposed** group of patients that are also investigated, and tends to recruit from a group of patients, rather than from a specific *population* of interest.

They are predominantly used to look at the natural history of an exposure.

Systematic review

Systematic reviews are **summaries of the literature**, performed by using explicit, reproducible methods of searching for, and critically appraising, available research. If the numerical results of included studies are combined to produce a single result, this is termed a 'meta-analysis'.

They have two key roles in medical research:
- Providing robust estimates of the effectiveness of an intervention, by using all good-quality available data.
- Identifying areas where research is lacking, so helping to direct future study.

Well-performed systematic reviews are considered the highest form of medical evidence.

Practice questions

1. What does the term 'level of evidence' mean?
    a. Broadly, describe the different levels of evidence.

2. For each of the following (i) describe how they're conducted; (ii) state strengths, weaknesses and common biases:
    a. Randomised controlled trial
    b. Cohort study
    c. Case-control study

3. What are the four phases of a randomised controlled trial?

4. What are some inherent issues with randomised controlled trials, when applied to surgery?

5. What is a systematic review and how is it conducted?
    a. What are the two key roles of a systematic review?

14.3.3: Patient-reported outcome measures

Patient-reported outcome measures (PROMs) are defined as **subjective measures** of health outcomes which are **reported by patients**. PROMs typically measure the functional status of a patient (or patient group) following an intervention, such as a surgical procedure or changes in a healthcare system.

Their utilisation in research has becoming increasingly common in recent decades, so a working knowledge of PROMs is helpful.

Surgeons will typically encounter PROMs as a measure of the effect of a surgical intervention. In this context, pre- and post-intervention surveys are completed by a patient and may be further repeated at pre-defined timepoints.

Key knowledge

PROMs entered widespread use in the NHS in the early 2000s to measure outcomes following core elective procedures. They are now used increasingly to:

- assess **service quality** and **quality improvement** interventions
- calculate **economic value** of treatments and systems
- understand the **patient value** of interventions
- quantify **disease burden** associated with conditions
- compare treatment options through a process of **audit** or **research**.

A range of tools are available with which to collect and quantify patient outcomes. These may be generic (assessing overall quality of health or life) or specific (assessing a particular body system, condition or intervention).

Health-related quality of life

Health-related quality of life (HRQoL) is considered a function of the interaction between biological, psychological, emotional and social factors. **HRQoL PROMs seek to measure overall quality of life and are therefore applicable to any individual or clinical situation**.

Their versatility allows the use of recognised, validated scoring systems in a wide range of settings, and scores can be compared freely with individuals in different groups or contexts. Common generic PROMS tools include:

- EuroQual-5D (EQ-5D)
- Medical Outcomes Study Short Form 36 (SF-36).

A drawback of generic quality of life PROMs, like those mentioned above, is their lack of specificity to a particular condition, patient group or situation. They may lack the sensitivity to detect important differences between patients within these groups. Specific PROM tools are employed to examine matters of health or function in particular settings, such as the limitations a patient feels as a result of a certain condition. Examples of disease- / system-specific PROM tools include:

- Disease of the Arm, Shoulder and Hand (QuickDASH)
- The Forgotten Joint Score
- Dermatology Quality of Life Index (DQLI).

Quality-adjusted life year

The quality-adjusted life year (QALY) is a measure of disease burden, which considers both the quality and the quantity of a life.

This measure is in widespread use in clinical research and is **most frequently seen in relation to economic analyses of healthcare interventions**.

> **Calculating a QALY score**
>
> - A QALY score is calculated by assigning a 'utility' value to a particular state of health and multiplying it by the years spent in that state.
> - QALY scores range from 1 (perfect health) to 0 (dead), and 1 QALY = 1 year of life in perfect health.
>   - N.B. it is possible to consider a health state to be 'worse than death', which is assigned a negative score.
> - A QALY curve can be produced which plots health-related quality of life on the y-axis against time on the x-axis.

A criticism often levelled at the QALY is that it represents an oversimplification of the advantages and disadvantages of a particular intervention. Patients' perceptions of their own wellbeing are variable, subjective and predicated on a complex biopsychosocial foundation. Furthermore, patients' judgements of the benefits, risks and other factors relating to a particular treatment are highly complex. Nonetheless, the QALY is a useful tool in the evaluation of cost–benefit decisions and remains in widespread use.

14.3.4: Research funding

Funding streams

Broadly, funding for research can be divided into **'commercial'** and **'non-commercial'**.

Commercial	The funding received from industry will often be for projects that are directly commercially relevant, so it is important that you understand where your research output would sit within the market.
	This is becoming an increasingly common funding stream, with arguments both for and against it (Gulbrandsen and Smeby, 2015)
Non-commercial	These bodies support the majority of science research funding in the UK and include:
	Charities • The Association of Medical Research Charities (AMRC) has >150 charity members who, collectively, fund ~40% of medical research in the UK. Of these charities, the Wellcome Trust is the largest and most well-known.

Government
- National Institute for Health Research (NIHR)
  - The NIHR is the largest single funder of health and care research in the UK.
  - It predominantly funds research that is directly applicable to the NHS, social care or public health.
  - It is funded by the Department of Health and Social Care.
- Research Councils (UK Research and Innovation; UKRI)
  - There are a number of 'research councils' in the UK; the Medical Research Council is the most relevant to healthcare.
  - Collectively, the 7 research councils are brought together by 'UK Research and Innovation (UKRI)', which aims to ensure that research and innovation flourish in the UK.
  - The UKRI is funded by the Department for Business, Energy and Industrial Strategy (BEIS) and is accountable to the Secretary of State. Consequently, funding received from the research councils is 'taxpayers' money'.
- UK Research Office (UKRO)
  - The UKRO is a subdivision of the UKRI that sits within the European Commission. Its purpose is to ensure that UK researchers can gain access to funding opportunities from EU-funded programmes and to support UK input into European research.

National academies
- The most relevant academy to healthcare is the Royal Society (RS).
- The RS is a society of scholars that promotes and funds research.
- They are largely funded by foundations / corporations / endowments, but also receive a grant from BEIS.

Internal funding
- Universities will often have funds that they have set aside for research. These typically include scholarships and fellowships.

The surgical interview

Over the course of a period of research, **it is common to receive multiple income streams from a number of different funders.**

Applying for funding

Applying for funding is often a time-intensive task and requires excellent planning, attention to detail and patience. Some of the keys to writing a successful application include:

1. **Preparation**
   a. Start looking for funding streams early; you require plenty of time to apply for funding.
   b. Read the specific requirements of the funding opportunity. You must ascertain your eligibility early to avoid wasting time.
   c. Understand how the money will be spent. This might include:
      i. materials
      ii. salary
      iii. travel
      iv. courses and conferences.
   d. Ask the funder questions if you are unclear on anything; it is better to ask early and correct your application.
   e. Seek advice from others who have gone through the process.

2. **Application**
   a. Ensure it's in the correct format; funders often have very exacting requirements on typeface, font size, line spacing, etc.
   b. Explain the:
      i. scientific interest and importance of the question
      ii. innovation
      iii. feasibility
      iv. impact
      v. value for money.
   c. Avoid jargon.
   d. Ensure it has been proofed by a number of people prior to submission.

References

BMA (2004) *Safe handover: safe patients*.

General Medical Council (2020a) *Ethical Guidance for Doctors – decision making and consent*. Available at: www.gmc-uk.org/ethical-guidance/ethical-guidance-for-doctors/decision-making-and-consent/the-seven-principles-of-decision-making-and-consent

General Medical Council (2020b) *Ethical Guidance for Doctors – leadership and management for all doctors*. Available at: www.gmc-uk.org/ethical-guidance/ethical-guidance-for-doctors/leadership-and-management-for-all-doctors/duties-of-a-doctor-in-the-workplace

General Medical Council (2020c) *Ethical Guidance for Doctors – raising and acting on concerns*. Available at: www.gmc-uk.org/ethical-guidance/ethical-guidance-for-doctors/raising-and-acting-on-concerns/about-this-guidance

Gulbrandsen, M. and Smeby, J-C. (2015) Industry funding and university professors' research performance. *Research Policy*, **34(6)**: 932–50.

Healthcare Improvement Scotland (2019) *Learning from adverse events through reporting and review: a national framework for Scotland*. Available at: www.healthcareimprovementscotland.org/his/idoc.ashx?docid=968c1d9d-7439-41d7-83d5-531afebaebcc&version=-1

NHS Improvement (2018) *Never Event List 2018*. Available at: www.england.nhs.uk/publication/never-events

Oxford Centre for Evidence-Based Medicine (2009) *Levels of Evidence*. Available at: www.cebm.net/2009/06/oxford-centre-evidence-based-medicine-levels-evidence-march-2009/

Song, J.W. and Chung, K.C. (2010) Observational studies: cohort and case-control studies. *Plast Reconstr Surg*, **126(6)**: 2234–42. Available at: https://journals.lww.com/plasreconsurg/Fulltext/2010/12000/Observational_Studies__Cohort_and_Case_Control.58.aspx

Wartolowska, K., Collins, G.S., Hopewell, S. *et al*. (2016) Feasibility of surgical randomised controlled trials with a placebo arm: a systematic review. *BMJ Open*, **6**: e010194. Available at: https://bmjopen.bmj.com/content/bmjopen/6/3/e010194.full.pdf

The surgical interview